Rainbow Dreaming

A Big Book of Calm

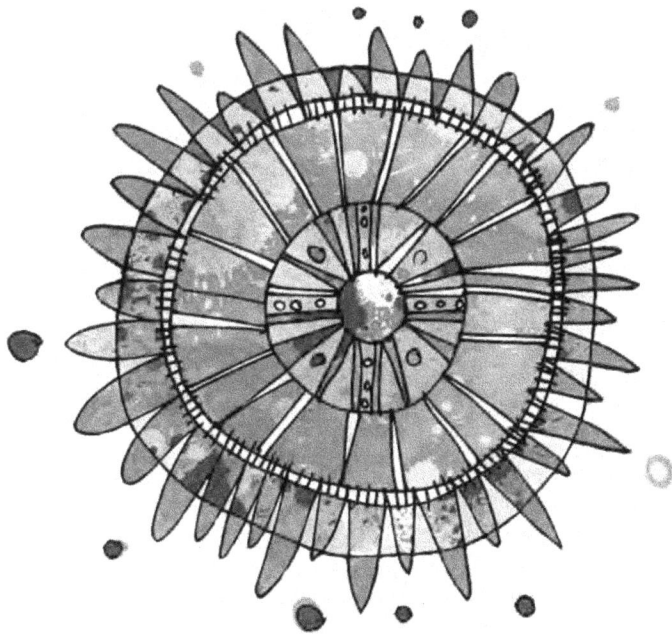

Amy Hamilton

All correspondence to the publisher
Indigo Kidz
PO Box 424
Floreat 6014
Western Australia

ISBN 978-0-9944546-0-7

Category: Health & Wellbeing: Self-Esteem: Meditation & Affirmations: Author: Title

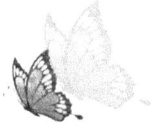

*For my husband and three beautiful children, the shining lights in my life
and for my brave mum who fought so hard to stay with us.*

With much love and thanks

To my brilliant and talented friend and artist, Kelly Jervis, you are the best.

To my friends and family, especially my aunt Sandra, who has let me bounce
ideas and listened to my endless ideas and rambling.

To all the teachers and parents who gave up their time to be interviewed and
who shared their knowledge, especially Deb Sewell - a true gem.

And finally in memory of Associate Professor, Ray James, who gave me a start
in the Health Promotion field and was always a gentle guiding hand throughout
my years of study. Thanks for sowing the meditation seed.

About the Author

Amy Hamilton lives in Western Australia with her husband and three children. Amy currently teaches in a secondary school and in her spare time she teaches meditation to children and writes resources and books to nurture children's spirituality. Amy has herself been practicing meditation for over 15 years and is passionate about it being introduced as part of the school curriculum. She also trains parents and teachers to teach meditation to children.

Amy Hamilton is a qualified secondary school teacher who has also worked in primary school and early childhood centres. Amy has a Diploma of Teaching, Bachelor of Education, Post Graduate Diploma of Health Promotion and a Masters Degree in Health Promotion. Amy is an accredited Children's Meditation Facilitator and is trained in Reiki, Children's Yoga and Crystal Therapy.

About the Artist

Kelly Jervis is a talented Sydney based illustrator artist and mother. Kelly's artistic background extends from set design and artistic installations to airbrushing and digital illustration. Kelly's amazing artwork features on all Indigo Kidz, Affirmation Garden and Rainbow Dreaming books and products and is available in a range of posters. Kelly is the Creative director and facilitator of the Kidzcollective Project. The project operates in primary schools and collaborates with students to create their own positive affirmation self portraits in line with their intentions. The project produces professional, contemporary digitally printed and mounted artworks for students and is creative, empowering and successful fundraising tool for schools. Kelly can be contacted at kidzcollective@gmail.com or visit her website at www.kidzcollectiveproject.com.au or like her Facebook page https://www.facebook.com/Kidzcollective.

Contents

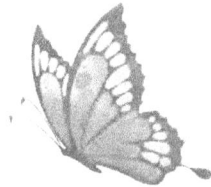

Happiness is a butterfly which, when pursued,

is always beyond our grasp, but which,

if you will sit down quietly,

may alight upon you.

Nathaniel Hawthorne

INTRODUCTION

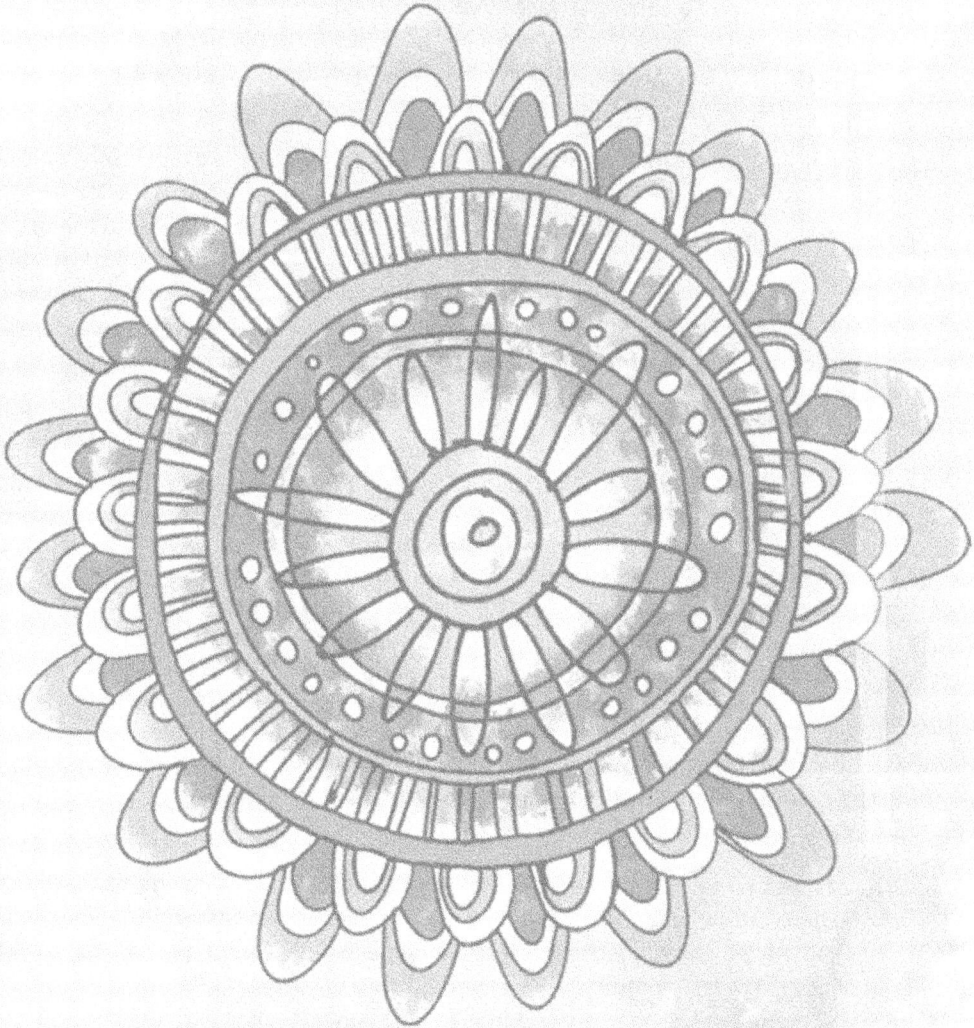

Author's Note

Since writing my first book *Indigo Dreaming* I have been asked many times how I started teaching meditation and relaxation to children, so I will share my story.

I was teaching health education in a secondary school during 1990 when I was timetabled to take a class of 15 year olds, who were, from all reports, *challenging*. The thought of staying home and hiding under my bed flitted across my mind many times as I wrestled with the problem of turning up to teach them.

I had tried many methods and ways to stimulate my class and provide a safe, friendly learning environment. I always had this particular class after lunch, which seemed to make them harder to motivate. One day I had the idea to teach them progressive muscle relaxation as part of the program. We moved the tables and chairs, did some deep breathing and followed a meditation cassette tape that I had come across in a shop. This was the start of a minor miracle. Not only did I have twenty five students (after initial giggles and wriggling) actually lying still, I had time to catch my breath. Quiet gently descended upon the class as they actually listened and participated in the process. I wondered if they had fallen asleep, then I would see the students' body parts tightening and relaxing as the voice on the tape directed.

After the progressive muscle relaxation the children moved back into their seats and I continued with our health education lesson. Suddenly, I found my class listening, quiet and interested. I continued to expand on this and introduce meditation using visualisation and focusing on the breath. I found the kids responded beyond my wildest dreams. They wanted to do it every lesson and the output afterwards was incredible.

During one lesson the Principal walked passed the classroom door and stopped to see what I was doing. He was astounded to discover that I had three of his most frequent visitors (not for good work, I might add) sitting quietly, participating and focusing on the class material. I am sure he initially thought that I had drugged them. It is also interesting to note that these students did not miss any health classes for the rest of the term. I had found a way to create a fantastic learning environment which they enjoyed and participated in.

It became very clear that I was teaching these students a much needed life-skill, how to take time to be still and focus and to be in the current moment. I needed no further convincing and this was the start of an incredible journey.

On a personal note as I was writing this second book my youngest son was having some difficulty reading and writing at school. After a few appointments and a visit to the Developmental Ophthalmologist he was diagnosed with X-linked Juvenile Retinoschisis. This is a genetic condition affecting boys which leads to becoming clinically blind. There is no medical cure as yet and the time line is unknown. My son has now lost almost 95% of his vision in the last 18 months and is now legally blind. Dealing with the condition and trying to find out more information has been a constant challenge and a path filled with many obstacles.

Initially we were devastated. I started to think about how it would change his life and the impact it would have on him and the family. He has had many things taken from his reach such as playing contact sports, driving a car and riding his bike out on the street. Yet I also realised that as a family we cannot get lost in a possible future but need to focus on all the things that he can do.

Our whole family has had to adjust. It is not just his vision that has been affected. His hearing has compensated by becoming much more acute, so big crowds and noise can overwhelm him. He has to concentrate and focus so much more at school now and often comes home completely exhausted, unreasonable and stressed. My older children have to assist him with certain tasks and we have had to make our house an obstacle-free zone so that he does not trip and fall.

Now more than ever I realise how important the process of visualisation and relaxation is going to be for us as a family. As my son's outer vision diminishes I am hoping that his inner vision is able to guide him. Differing methods of relaxation and calming techniques are part of his daily routine so that he can cope with the extra demands on his body and to help him deal with the changes.

The unknown is always in the back of my mind, but I can honestly say that meditation and calming techniques are helping greatly and without the tools in this book, our family and my son would not be coping as well as we are. He is growing into a confident, happy young boy who is taking everything in his stride.

Imagine someone told you that there is a way
to help a child to be happy, balanced and relaxed.

That they would sleep more deeply, be focused
and have greater concentration at school.

In addition, they would be better equipped to
deal with stress and that this 'way'
was fun and that they would enjoy it.

What would you be prepared to pay?

What if you were then told that it is free and easy
and could be done anywhere at any time
and only took a few minutes of your time?

Would you be interested?

Then read on...

New Shoes

How our Grandparents Shopped:

I needed a new pair of shoes and decided that today would be a good day to look for them. I had jobs to do but they could wait. My daughter and I decided to catch the train as it was such a nice day. We walked to the train station enjoying the fresh air. My daughter paid for our ticket at the machine and made sure we had the correct one for the number of zones we were travelling through.

When the train arrived we found a seat and set off for the shops. We pronounced and counted all the train stops on the way. We watched as all the different people got on and off. My daughter and I stood up when an elderly couple got on and enjoyed the rest of the ride standing up. We arrived at the shops taking in all the sights and smells. We walked through shops, up and down stairs and escalators trying to find ones that I liked. We tried on at least a dozen pairs discussing the merits of each one before we found a pair we both liked. We thanked the sales assistant, and as we left the shop we noticed that the delicious fragrance of the cakes, bread and rolls in the bakery was just too good to pass by. We nibbled on our morning tea and listened with enchantment as a busker played his guitar. We walked back towards the train station and ran into an old friend that we had not seen in many years. It was great to see her and find out how her family was doing. We caught the train back home enjoying the ride as it gently rocked along the tracks. We walked back home carrying our newly purchased shoes chatting along the way. What a great way to spend the day...

How we Shop Today:

I needed a new pair of shoes. I went online. I used an app to search for the pair I liked and got them at the lowest price possible. I showed them to my daughter and she said they were nice. I paid by credit card and they will be delivered to my door within 48 hours.

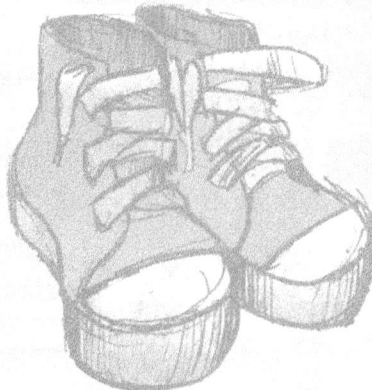

Introduction

Our modern word is fast-paced and stress filled. Technology continues to advance at breath-taking speed and it seems that our society values how much we can produce in a short amount of time. Technology has made some incredible advances and will continue to do so. I want to stress that I am not anti-technology however, I believe we need to ask ourselves just how this fast-paced environment is affecting our children and various aspects of their growth and development.

Childhood health statistics, around the world, paint an unpleasant picture of increasing obesity, mental health issues, phobias, obsessive compulsive disorders, depression, ADHD, ADD, autism, poor body image, aggression, teenage suicide, cancers, diabetes and the list goes on. Add to this the latest research suggesting that up to 20 percent of children do not sleep properly and/or get enough sleep and it gets worse. We need to ask ourselves if our modern environment and all this marvellous technology is contributing to increased behavioural, developmental, mental health and social problems.

Our amazing new technology offers us instant results and that which must be waited for is suddenly deemed "slow" and "old fashioned." It seems we are becoming a society of instant gratification and patience, perseverance, and stead-fast resolve have become outdated. You only have to turn on the television news report to hear about yet another road rage incident. There are so many innovative ideas that promise to make life easier and save us precious time, yet so many of us are stressed and always running out of time. This begs the question: With all these "time saving" devices, why are so many adults and children suffering from stress related diseases and ailments?

We run from meeting to meeting and rush from one activity to another. We talk on phones, on computers and in cars. We are working longer hours and are accessible to our work 24 hours a day. You go to a cafe for lunch and mobile phones are ringing, people are talking on their phones or playing with some form of electronic device, no standing in a queue quietly anymore and being on your own when out is not an issue if you have your device with you. As soon as we buy an electronic product there seems to be an update or new 'app' so we all rush to get the new one thus discarding the now antique-like version. Are we as a society becoming addicted to speed? What happens if we can't keep up or if things are not fast enough for us? Perhaps we get frustrated, stressed, or angry. We may then act out of character or in an aggressive manner. Does this sound familiar?

We can shop online, date online, have friends and do business online. We hold major meetings over video conferencing. The internet has become another "virtual" member of our social group so if you want to read a book or the news you can download it instantly. Even our language is faster. We use abbreviations and acronyms to make our messaging quicker. Is our convenient instant existence robbing our children of valuable experiences and life lessons? How often do we hear children say, "I am bored" if they have to sit still with no television, computers or other forms of external stimulation. This boredom can result in children misbehaving or becoming overly active. Children expect to be entertained and it seems parents are expected to be constantly on their toes to provide it.

We have media and technological applications that are mind boggling. We marvel at the amazing special effects used in movies and the imaginary worlds of computer games. Televisions are now in 3D and almost all children's movies are now in 3D. Our children are constantly bombarded with many different stimuli as well as exposure to content that is age inappropriate, overtly sexual and violent. A child's developing brain is now forced to process millions of pieces of information daily, something our ancestors never, ever experienced.

Along with our incredibly rapid pace of life comes the fast-food and ready-to-eat meals. We have nutrition snack-bars and sports drinks that the advertisers say help to give kids energy and keep them alert. Bottled water has somehow become one of the biggest money-makers for manufacturers whilst causing huge environmental issues. We don't seem to have time to prepare and cook as we used to. Now we have cookbooks touting fast and easy meals, usually using minimal ingredients or pre-prepared sauces, simply flying off the shelves.

Research suggests children are spending huge amounts of time indoors watching television, using computers and electronic devices. We are more disconnected from the outdoors and from nature than our parents and grandparents before us. Technology such as social network sites and social media applications enables our children to keep in touch with friends, to express themselves, be creative, to share photos as well as organise events. However they also enable our children's lives to be displayed in public like never before. They know immediately if they are not invited to an event. They have physical and public proof if someone won't be their friend on Facebook or has deleted them as a friend. Social networks can be invasive and with their introduction and popularity we have a new set of problems. Bullying is not a new issue, but cyber-bullying, leading to new legislation and awareness campaigns to combat it, is. Some children find making virtual friends easier than communicating and socialising in real life. Reality shows dominate our television screens further fuelling the invasiveness of our culture.

Parents are equally under stress. We face stress at work, as well as stress from trying to keep up with the modern ideal of being a success. The days where mum stayed home and dad worked are all but gone for the majority of the population. Both parents often work. Today we see single and blended families, children living with grandparents, children in foster care and so on. Family structures are changing rapidly. Parents are working longer hours and many children are spending a substantial amount of time in day care or other forms of care. Many grandparents are being called on to help raise their grandchildren while their children work.

It seems that having "stuff" is just part of modern culture. Our love of material things is evident by national sales figures and our soaring personal debt. Often our children have mobile phones, iPhones, iPads and credit cards before they even have a full-time job. Our current generation of parents have been part of the compulsive consumerism that has swept through the world. Having "stuff" makes you happy, according to the advertisers. In fact we often use the term "retail therapy" to justify this excessive spending on luxury and non-essential items. So if "retail therapy" works, why are depression rates so high? Why do we have an epidemic of unhappy, unhealthy adults and unhappy, unhealthy children? The additional stresses to low-income families include hunger, lack of accommodation and violence as well as emotions centred around not being a "success" in the eyes of our society.

The place we call home is also changing. Houses are getting bigger and backyards smaller. We now need media rooms, outdoor rooms, three or four bathrooms, several toilets and of course parents must have their own retreat! Many new housing designs offer only a small courtyard as an outdoor garden. So often they are impersonal little concrete cells.

The schooling system is left-brain orientated. Children are not taught how to focus or concentrate. They are just expected to do this automatically with only minimal amounts of education devoted to helping children understand themselves and learning to access their own inner skills. This is not the fault of teachers who may be overwhelmed with an extensive curriculum, reporting demands, large class sizes and increases in pupils with learning difficulties and behavioural problems within their classrooms. All the knowledge in the world is of no use if we don't understand how our thoughts and emotions affect us. Emotions and thoughts help shape our behaviour and who we become. An understanding of emotions and thoughts also helps us to prepare for learning.

Children today often live a frenetic lifestyle. Parents are constantly hurrying to get children to their extra-curricular commitments. Young children are often rushed off to day care early in the morning. Older children attend regular school, and are often enrolled in extracurricular activities or after school day care. In addition they have homework and then somewhere in between they fit in sleep and eating. I am not saying that after school activities are not of benefit, generally they are of great value and children respond well to scheduled activity and structure. However as parents and educators we have to ask if these extra-curricular activities benefit the child or society's expectations? Perhaps children just need some downtime to learn how to process their day and enable their body to respond accordingly.

When do children actually relax? When do they have time to just "be"? Where are they taught how to be calm, centred and focused? If we can help children to slow down and enjoy being still, we may be able to help them find the answers internally instead of looking to the external for happiness and stimulation. We can teach children to look within when they are stressed and anxious, to help them find their own sense of peace and tranquillity rather than reacting to what is going on around them. This fast-paced world is not going to slow down but our children need to be taught that they don't have to be entrapped into being busy all the time. Children need time to reflect and re-energise so they can meet the challenges that life offers.

Teaching children relaxation, calming strategies and basic meditation through visualisation can help young children cope with their emotions and thought processes. They learn to understand themselves better when they take the time to sit quietly and to be still. They learn to just "be". They can learn to recognise if they are stressed and how to counteract it. I believe our children are evolving more rapidly than we realise and so may require different educational processes and approaches. By learning to take the time to sit and be still they will also get a better appreciation of what is going on around them and perhaps see things more clearly.

The term Meditation can be easily misunderstood. There are many different types of beliefs and customs associated with different schools of religion and philosophy and they all have their rich traditions. I teach what I believe works well with children and is of most benefit to them at this young age.

I teach relaxation and meditation to children in a practical, simple way without any religious beliefs or the use of confusing jargon. I present a format that I hope parents and teachers can easily relate to and understand. I suggest that this system can be a stepping stone towards discovering how enjoyable and how easy teaching relaxation and meditation to children can be.

I hope that one day relaxation and meditation will be part of a daily routine for all school-aged children. Teaching relaxation and meditation is effective, cost efficient and readily accessible. Peaceful, happy and contented children become peaceful, happy and contented adults. The basic skills of meditation and relaxation enable children to tap into their own internal calm, their creativity and strengths.

There is more to life than increasing its speed.
Mahatma Gandhi

About Rainbow Dreaming

Why Rainbows?

Colours are around us everywhere. We see them in nature, in what we eat and drink, our clothes, our shoes and our homes. Colours can change moods, evoke feelings and emotions and can even affect our behaviour. Arguably one of nature's most impressive displays of colour effects is the rainbow. Children love the magic of rainbows.

Rainbow Dreaming continues on from the introductory book, *Indigo Dreaming,* and revises and updates current teaching methods. It introduces the concept of colour and its energetic healing properties. It explores meditation and relaxation with children more deeply. *Rainbow Dreaming* uses the seven traditional colours of the rainbow to provide over 50 new visualisations and more wonderful adventures and activities for children to enjoy.

Visualisations

The visualisations in *Rainbow Dreaming* are separated under each colour of the rainbow with each section focusing on different key issues or values. The visualisations in this book encourage children to explore their emotions and their imaginations. Children can discover things about themselves and the way they relate to others. They can explore places and do things that may not be possible in everyday life. The visualisations instil important life qualities and explore key values such as compassion and gratitude. They allow children to be creative and to use their minds without external stimulation. Some of the visualisations in the book take the child on an external journey of adventure and some will take them on an internal journey allowing the opportunity to look within and discover that quiet place we all have inside.

Affirmations are included with each visualisation to reinforce positive self talk. Each visualisation has a set of rainbow thoughts to prompt further discussion or for use in a sharing circle.

The visualisations listed under the *Rainbow* section tend to be slightly longer and focus predominantly on achieving balance.

Who can Use this Book?

The book is predominantly aimed at primary school aged children but can be enjoyed by anyone of any age. Parents, grandparents, guardians, caregivers, teachers and health professionals can use this book. It can be used in a class setting, at home or for one-on-one counselling sessions. The visualisations are also great to use in children's yoga and massage classes.

Special Features

For ease of reading, I have referred to parent/teacher or child/children throughout the text. *Italics* have been used for all spoken parts in the meditation to alert the reader and to enable the meditation to flow. All references and research documents are listed at the back and not placed throughout the book.

In response to requests I have included some experiences from parents and teachers and suggested meditation outlines. I have also listed some of my favourite resources that I use when teaching in schools and with my own children.

There is an index of meditations and key values to make the visualisations easy to find.

I hope you and your children enjoy the new adventures and I encourage all parents and teachers who do not meditate or practice any form of relaxation to try it and discover the benefits for yourself.

Being

relaxed and calm

can be contagious!!

What Children can Learn from this Book

- Understand that breathing affects their energy levels and is a simple way to change the way they feel.
- Being aware of their body and how it can affect their feelings and emotions.
- How they react to external influences and the effects it can have on their body.
- To recognise the signs and symptoms that their body is under stress.
- To use visualisation and meditation to turn on their relaxation response, and to manage their emotions and feelings in a positive way.
- To use positive self talk and positive thoughts to creative a positive attitude towards themselves and life.
- To develop an attitude of gratitude.
- To be mindful in all aspects of life.
- To believe in themselves and trust their inner wisdom.
- To use their imagination and tap into their creativity each and every day.
- To understand that colours can help balance, change moods and energy levels.
- To have a large and varied tool kit of strategies to keep calm, confident, happy and creative in our fast paced world.
- To understand that we all have a place of quiet within us that we can access at any time.
- That it is ok to just "be".

* * * * * * *

Welcome to the world of

Rainbow Dreaming

STRESS IN CHILDREN

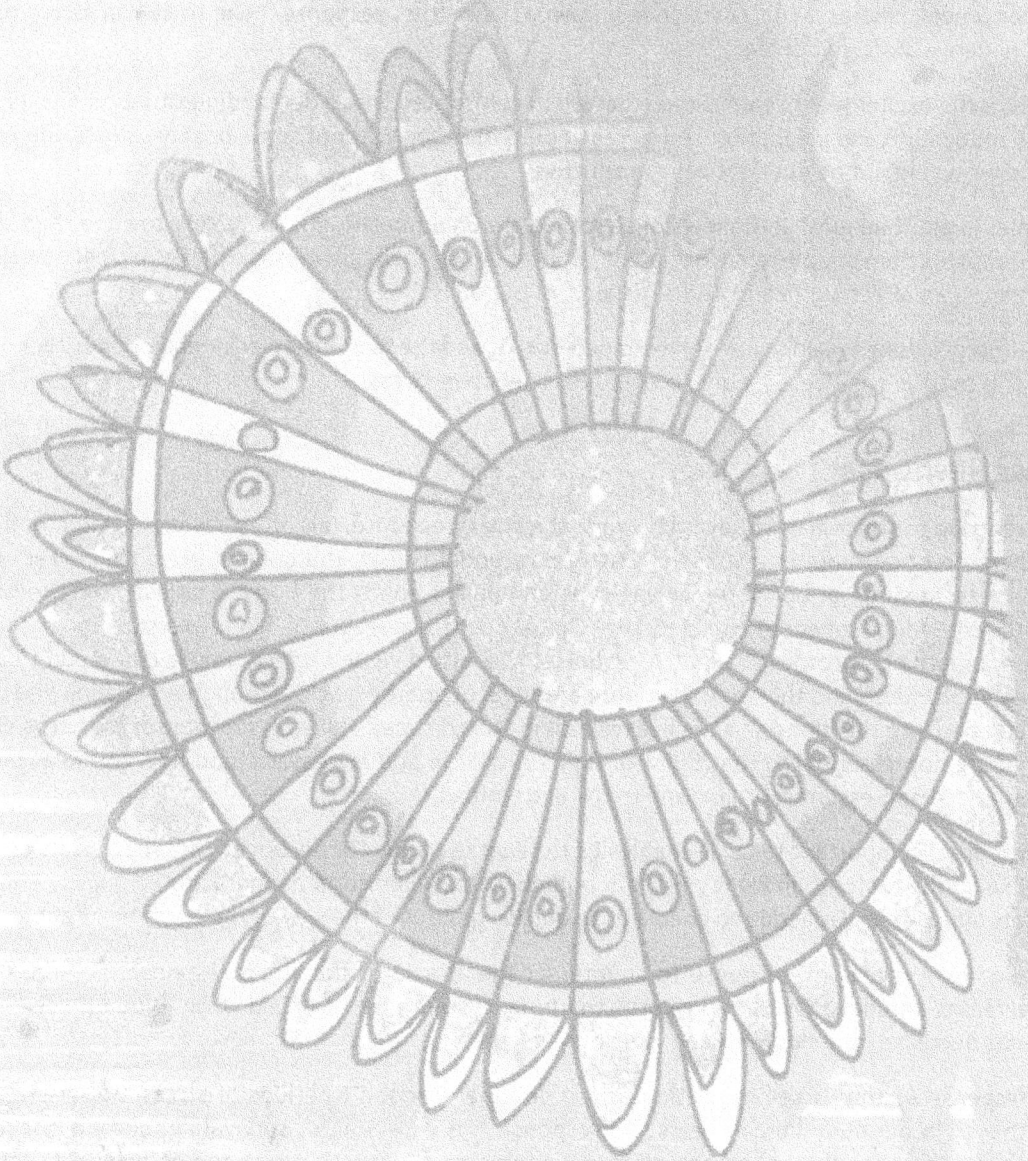

What is Stress?

Stress is one of those words that are bandied around. Simply put, everyone has stress in their lives to some extent, everyday. We can't live without stress. Stress is the normal response to a stressor, a situation or event that causes or provokes stress. This reaction is known as our stress response. I like to talk in terms of the positive and negative stress in our life.

Positive stress is the excitement or thrill people get when confronted with a demanding situation or events. It helps us with motivation and inspiration and to reach our potential. Without some positive stress, life would be boring and we would not be as effective or productive.

Negative stress is the "bad guy." If the level of stress we are under outweighs our ability to cope then stress becomes a problem. Often people refer to it as being "stressed out". Negative stress makes us feel unwell and uncomfortable. It can affect our health and all aspects of our daily life.

How stress affects us depends upon our ability to deal with it and the resources we are equipped with. For the purposes of this chapter the stress we are referring to is negative stress.

The Stress Response

The natural reaction to stress in the body is known as the stress response. It is often called the "fight or flight" reaction. When the body is put in a stressful situation or under threat, the brain starts a chain reaction in the body that sees a surge of hormones released as adrenaline floods the body. It adjusts metabolism to allow a greater expenditure of energy to take place. During the stress-response, blood pressure and breathing rates increase, breathing becomes shallow, digestion slows, blood vessels widen, pupils dilate and muscles tighten. Sweat is produced and the body uses large amounts of energy quickly through adrenaline and other hormones releasing into the blood and the liver releasing stored sugar. The stress response also curbs bodily functions that are non-essential to the "flight or fight" response and increases blood flow to major organs while decreases it to non-essential organs and to the extremities.

The stress response is important to us. It enables us to react to danger or perceived threats. If, for example, we see a snake on the footpath in front of us, our body becomes alerted to danger and the quickly released hormones sets off a physical reaction to enable us to quickly get out of the way of the perceived danger.

The body also has a relaxation response to counteract the affects of the stress response. The relaxation response decreases adrenalin levels and returns the body system to a balanced state. Blood pressure and breathing rates decrease, muscles relax and digestion resumes.

Our stress response system is self-regulating and is designed for short periods of stress, not continuous, prolonged stress. In our early human years this response was essential for survival i.e. getting out of the way of predators. After the threat had passed, and we felt safe and secure again, the body would naturally return to its normal functioning state. In our modern environment, stress is more likely caused by rapid social change and the pressures placed upon us. Expectations are high, lifestyles are getting more sedentary and everything, including our food, is fast. With modern technology we often have difficulties switching off from our work life, we are accessible all the time. Our new predators include beasts such as cyber bullying, living up to expectations, relationship difficulties and lack of money. We often create threats and pressure through our own perceptions of how our life should look. Because of this, our body's stress response is being activated for long periods of time or is failing to turn off at all. The perceived threat or predator constantly surrounds us. This constant, and unrelenting level of stress is therefore becoming harmful to our systems, causing damage to our cells and organs and directly affecting our immune system. Of course, over time, this onslaught leads to disease and illness.

Stress response does not turn off = Body organs and cells affected
Changes in our body's ability to function = Symptoms & Disease

It seems we are getting so used to the constant stress facing us that we think it is normal to feel this way. Children especially may be unaware that they are in a state of stress which is why it is important to teach them the signs and symptoms and simple ways to counteract stress. Perhaps some of the diagnoses we are seeing for childhood disorders such as ADHD and depression are actually related to the child's stress level and the inability to switch off the stress response system.

Food for Thought

It is very interesting to note that current research in the field of *Evolutionary Health Promotion* suggests that our genes may be mismatched to the current environment in which we live. It suggests genes that predispose us to illness may have been selected to suit certain environmental pressures and that technology has advanced so quickly that our bodies have not had time to adapt. Studies of primitive people show that they appear to be almost free of chronic degenerative diseases. Interestingly, chronically degenerative diseases, which generally produce mortality later in life, begin in childhood.

Stress in Children

As discussed, stress in its negative form has a profound effect on a person's wellbeing. Studies indicate that stress is the underlying cause of the majority of diseases. It has been linked to: hypertension, heart attacks, diabetes, asthma, allergies, chronic pain, headaches, backaches, skin disorders, cancer, compromised immune systems, decrease in white blood cells, ulcers, changes in white blood cells, weight problems, arthritis and depression, to list a few.

With childhood depression, asthma, diabetes, obesity and cancer rates increasing world-wide, it is vital that parents and teachers understand stress and the body's response to it. Only then can we appreciate how vital the benefits of meditation and other calming techniques are for children.

What Causes Stress in Children?

The causes of stress in children are wide and varying. Stress affects everyone in different ways. What may seem insignificant to an adult can be of major consequence to a child. What may be mildly challenging to one child can cause another to have a complete meltdown. Some children experience upsets such as fighting with a sibling or doing homework whilst others may face upsets that include physical, sexual or verbal abuse. Some children face the stress of trying to find food and shelter as part of their daily life.

Children's temperaments, personalities and natural resilience can affect how they react to stress. Children can manifest similar stress symptoms to adults but may deal with it differently. Often we dismiss stress in children and it is put down to other childhood ailments such as tiredness or illness, when in fact they are stressed. Children don't always understand their symptoms and misread the signs of stress. Instead of being able to recognise stress, they act out and react with behaviours such as aggression and being naughty. Some children do not know how to verbalise or express how they are feeling. They are either too young or have not developed the skills or confidence.

As a teacher I have seen the incidence of behavioural problems, learning disorders and syndromes increase rapidly in the last 20 years. Go back another 15 odd years to when I attended primary school and I can remember one child in our class who had a few behavioural issues. I am not saying that these conditions do not exist or that they are not valid, but I wonder if all the children that are diagnosed with a variety of disorders and labels actually have them. Perhaps they are just reacting to that fact that they are extremely stressed, over stimulated and completely out of balance.

As a society we have a pill for every ill and medicating children is often done as a first resort not as a last. It has become a form of behaviour management in some cases and teaches children that drugs are a coping mechanism. Again I understand that some children require medication and have some very serious issues that require expert medical attention and professional intervention, however could we not also teach them self coping skills? Teaching a child relaxation and meditation can only benefit other strategies that are in place.

Symptoms of Stress in Children

When a child is stressed they may exhibit both physical and emotional symptoms. It is important that adults and teachers recognise that a child's behaviour may be a result of stress, anxiety or panic. As parents and teachers we need to be observant and not misinterpret children's signals and behaviour. We need to be aware of changes in a child's behaviour so that if they are under stress it can be properly managed. Young children often do not have the ability to understand that the "bad" feeling may be because of stress let alone be able to express it. Trust your instincts; if you observe changes in a child's behaviour then act on it.

Some of the Physical Symptoms:
- Headaches
- Feeling sick
- Stomach pain
- Sore muscles
- Diarrhoea or constipation
- Indigestion
- Loss of appetite or overeating
- Inability to sleep/nightmares
- Inability to concentrate
- Increased heart rate
- Poor memory
- Breathing difficulties
- Bed wetting
- Lethargy

Some of the Emotional Symptoms:
- Nervousness
- Anxiety
- Sadness, crying, tearful
- Aggression, irritability and anger
- Bullying others
- Tension
- Fidgeting
- Moody, negative thoughts
- Lacking confidence/ low self-esteem
- Withdrawal
- Attention seeking behaviours
- Clingy behaviour
- Naughty Behaviour/ tantrums
- Not wanting to go to school

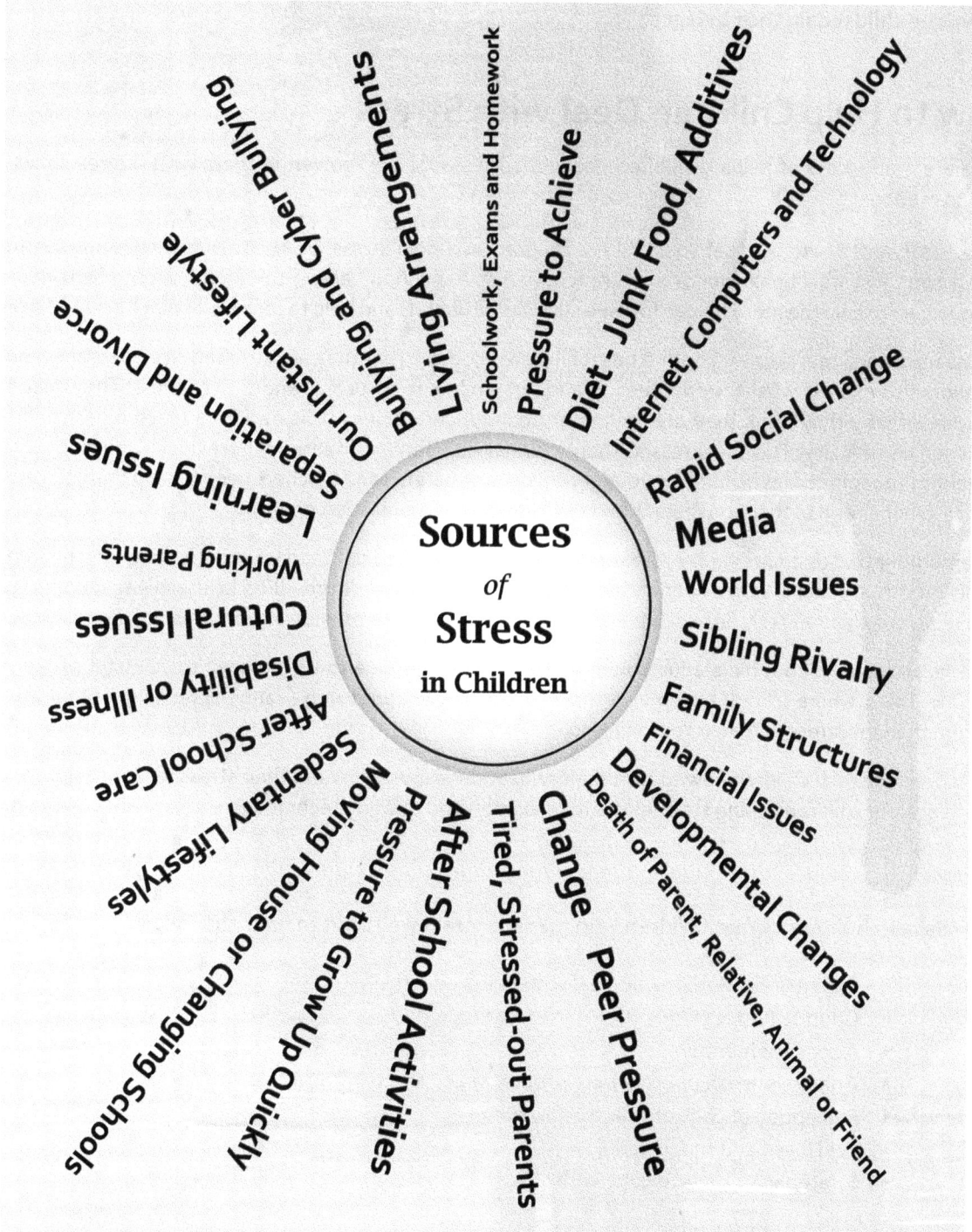

Sources *of* Stress in Children

- Living Arrangements
- Schoolwork, Exams and Homework
- Pressure to Achieve
- Diet - Junk Food, Additives
- Internet, Computers and Technology
- Rapid Social Change
- Media
- World Issues
- Sibling Rivalry
- Family Structures
- Financial Issues
- Developmental Changes
- Death of Parent, Relative, Animal or Friend
- Peer Pressure
- Change
- Tired, Stressed-out Parents
- After School Activities
- Pressure to Grow Up Quickly
- Moving House or Changing Schools
- Sedentary Lifestyles
- After School Care
- Disability or Illness
- Cultural Issues
- Working Parents
- Learning Issues
- Separation and Divorce
- Our Instant Lifestyle
- Bullying and Cyber Bullying

*** If you believe a child is suffering from chronic stress and displaying extreme symptoms of behaviour then they should be referred to medical professionals who can work together with parents and teachers to help the child regain their balance.

How to Help Children Deal with Stress

There are many ways of helping children deal with stress while empowering them with the resources they need to manage it.

- Be observant! Recognise that your child or children are under stress. Be aware of the signs and symptoms and don't just label behaviour or a child's reaction as a childhood ailment or inappropriate behaviour. The more we observe the more we can foresee stressful situations and help to remove or block a child's stressor.

- As parents and teachers we need to help children recognise that they are stressed. We need to encourage children to express what they are feeling and put a name to it such as anger or sadness. They need to be aware of why they think they are feeling or acting a certain way. It is easier to teach older children to recognise that they may be stressed than younger children. As mentioned previously, putting words to feelings can sometimes be hard for younger children so parents and teachers need to help them to verbalise their feelings and to manage them. Keep the lines of communication open.

- Remember that as adults we are role-models. If we are stressed out then we are teaching our children that this is normal behaviour. We need to be calm, positive role models providing love and engagement whilst making our children feel safe, secure and reassured. We need to provide a supportive environment.

- Some children will not have adult role models and will continue to be exposed to stressful situations at home. This is where schools become so important arming children with a range of techniques that will help them manage stress and their responses to it.

- We need to teach children how to turn their relaxation response on and their stress response off. We need to teach our children coping strategies and relaxation and calming techniques.

Research shows us that Children who manage stress well tend to have the following:

- Parents/role Models who deal with stress effectively
- Good self esteem
- A sense of humour
- Good relationships with friends, parents and teachers
- Perception of control over their lives
- Feel loved and supported
- Strategies or tools to cope with stress

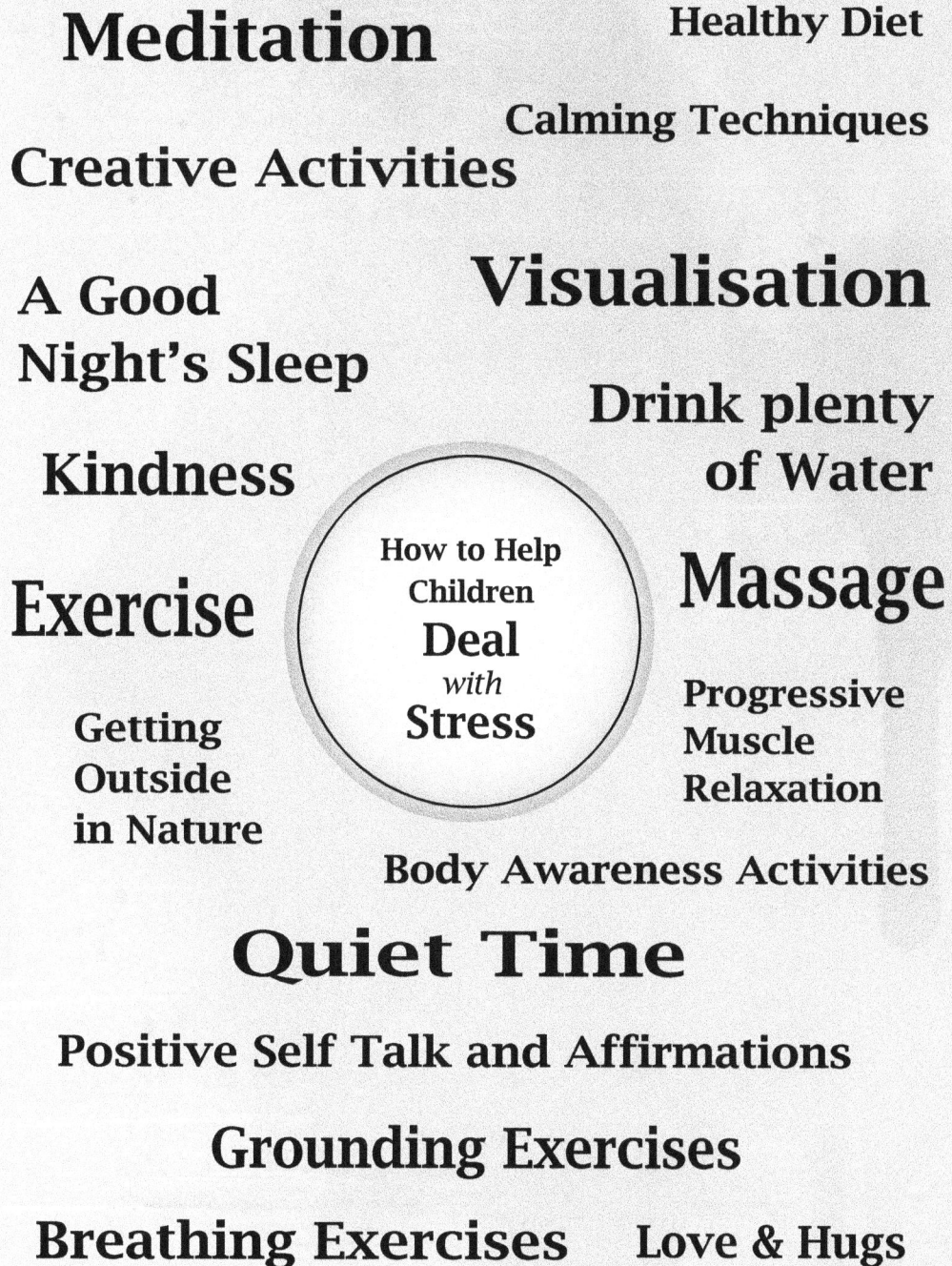

Meditation

Healthy Diet

Calming Techniques

Creative Activities

A Good
Night's Sleep

Visualisation

Drink plenty
of Water

Kindness

How to Help
Children
Deal
with
Stress

Massage

Exercise

Progressive
Muscle
Relaxation

Getting
Outside
in Nature

Body Awareness Activities

Quiet Time

Positive Self Talk and Affirmations

Grounding Exercises

Breathing Exercises   Love & Hugs

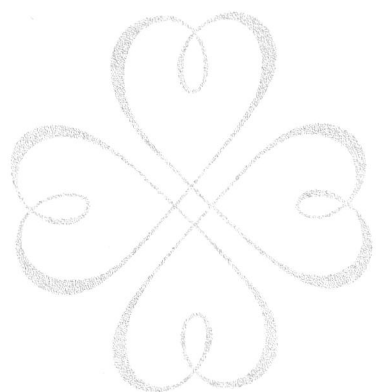

ABOUT MEDITATION AND RELAXATION

Tolerance Vitality Resilience
High Self Esteem Security
Passion for Life Freedom
Opportunities Fit & Healthy
Appreciation of Life Peace
Vitality   Empathy
Joy   Love

What Do We
Want
for our
Children?

Calm   Friends
Honesty   Respect
Curiosity   Gratitude
Empowerment Coping Skills
Kindness Compassion
Cultural Awareness
Fulfilling Relationships
Feeling of Connection

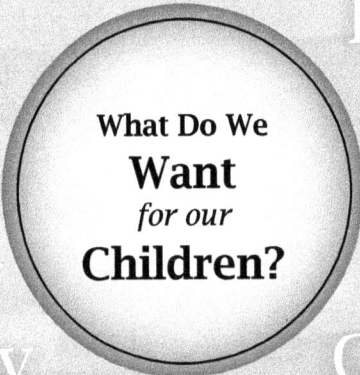

About Meditation and Relaxation with Children

What is Relaxation?

Relaxation, in a general sense, means releasing tension and returning the body to a state of balance or equilibrium. A relaxation technique is any activity, method, process or procedure that helps a person to relax or attain a state of calmness. Meditation is widely used as a relaxation technique.

What is Meditation?

Meditation is often over-defined, confusing and seems to encompass a whole range of techniques and practices. Meditation means different things to different people and sometimes a definition can be limiting. It is worthwhile exploring your own definition of the word meditation, what it means to you and why you think it is important for children to practice it. You can then share your ideas with your class or children.

When I discuss the term "meditation", I like to offer the following points.

- Meditation can be thought of as the calming and quietening of the mind, body, feelings and thoughts.
- It is a process that helps to foster the growth of the mind and body connection of the child and teaches children self-awareness and supports creativity.
- It teaches children to enjoy being still in the present moment and to focus their mind without mental chatter or distractions.
- Meditation is a unique physiological state which is different from sleep or ordinary wakefulness. The body enters a state of relaxation but at the same time, is alert.

In simple terms for a young child, meditation can be discussed as relaxing the body and calming the mind to make you feel better. Meditation helps children to find a safe quiet sanctuary within their mind. You can discuss that meditation is *"my time"*. It is a quiet time when you can listen to your thoughts and feelings and enjoy getting to know your inner-self better. I have heard a teacher explain to her young class that it is like "exercising the brain" and another teacher suggests that meditation is a way to make you feel completely happy, inside and out and to listen to your heart.

When working with children I like to encourage children to come up with their own definition of the word meditation. My daughter made herself a meditation book and in it she wrote, *"When you meditate, you close your eyes and your fingers, you relax, and then you imagine"*. Another child wrote, *"Meditation is my own special time to be quiet so that I can hear my heart talk to me"*. Children make it so simple!

What Meditation is Not!

Meditation is not daydreaming nor is it only done as part of a cult. It is not lots of happy wandering thoughts and it is not a form of brain-washing. You will not sprout mung beans from your ears nor will hundreds of animals and insects start following you when you walk down the street. You do not have to sit still for hours on a mountain in one position chanting. Meditation does not exclusively belong to any one philosophy or religion. Anyone, anywhere, of any background, any religion or belief can meditate and enjoy the benefits.

Why Meditate?

People meditate for many different reasons. Some people meditate to manage stress, some to enhance creativity, others to overcome personal issues, to improve health, or to get more in tune with themselves. The reasons are endless. Everyone can meditate and no matter what the reason, the benefits are universal.

Teaching children to meditate helps them to understand that they have the power to control their thoughts and emotions and that security lies within. Meditation can assist children to take responsibility for their actions and help them to redirect their energies in a more positive manner. It can help children cope with stress and create an optimal frame of mind for learning.

The Benefits of Meditation for Children

Benefits of Meditation

There are many benefits from regularly practicing meditation. These benefits affect the physical, mental, emotional and spiritual well being of a child. Abundant anecdotal research, coupled with scientific research, is now validating the fact that the mind-body connection to our overall well-being is far reaching.

Transcendental Meditation (TM), which became very popular in the 1960s, claims to be the most effective form of meditation and has over 500 research papers published on its effectiveness on the many aspects of human physiology and psychology. Dr Herbert Benson, an Associate Professor of Medicine at Harvard Medical School and founder of the Mind/Body Institute, has produced some groundbreaking scientific research in the areas of stress, relaxation and meditation. Michael Murphy and Steven Donavon from the Institute of Noetic Science have summarised hundreds of research studies, which discuss and analyse the physiological and psychological benefits of meditation.

Meditation has been linked to lowering blood pressure, boosting the immune system, lowering the heart rate, reducing muscle tension, aiding in the treatment of cancer and asthma, increasing cortical thickness, improved sleep, improving perceptual motor skills, decreasing anxiety, aggression and pain management and the list goes on.

In simple terms, here are some of the major benefits of meditation relevant to children;

- It encourages a healthy mind, body and spirit
- It encourages creativity and use of the imagination
- Children are less likely to have nightmares or bad dreams
- Children sleep better
- Helps children to balance their excess energy
- Provides a chance to re-energise
- It increases confidence and self-awareness
- It increases memory, focus and concentration
- It increases the ability to cope with stress
- It increases listening skills
- It develops positive attitudes

- It teaches relaxation skills and how to quiet the mind
- It helps to develop a sense of inner peace
- It provides children with a tool they will have for life
- It helps children to deal with emotions, thoughts and feelings which they may not fully understand
- It teaches children to enjoy time alone in a positive way
- It helps children to learn more effectively
- In our changing world, it teaches our children to use their minds without external stimulation

Meditation can positively affect all the physical and emotional symptoms of stress. It is interesting to note that many Government Health Agencies list meditation as a source of relaxation and a way to deal with stress on their websites and in their literature for the community, yet it is a skill not readily taught to our children.

Note: See references and articles in the Research section on our website
www.indigokidz.com.au

Creating an Optimal Learning Environment

Meditation has been long favoured for its health benefits but it can also compliment the process of learning. Children learn more effectively and absorb more information when they are relaxed and focused. If meditation can help produce this relaxed and focused state then surely it is of great benefit to the education system? How often do you hear teachers say that a child does not concentrate in class or does not focus on the task at hand? I have, myself, written similar comments on school reports in the past.

Our children are evolving much faster than previous generations. With the number of children now diagnosed with learning difficulties, it is time to further explore multi- sensory learning and the relationship between the left and right side of the brain, as well as whole brain learning. It seems children who are left-brained dominant are currently more suited to our education system. It may be that our current education system is far too linear and we now have more children who need to learn using alternate methods. Meditation may assist with this process. This is discussed further in the chapter *Meditation in Schools.*

A recent study into the effects of relaxation and visualisation on 5th grade students in Virginia, USA, found that relaxation and visualisation are effective study techniques. It summarised that students had an increased attention span and learned more effectively. The study went on to recommend that it be incorporated into all teacher training programs.

Alpha and Beta

When we are thinking and going about our daily lives, the brain emits Beta brain waves. This is the normal state of consciousness that we operate in for most of the day. Beta is a state of thinking and doing and at some point, if we do too much thinking and doing, our energy levels drop and we get tired. Over stimulation and too much stress can tire children rather quickly.

When we relax, the electrical activity of the brain, or brain waves, change and become, bigger, slower and more rhythmical. These patterns are called Alpha brain waves. Alpha helps us to create scenes and images in our mind allowing us to sense and feel things more clearly. Operating in Alpha rejuvenates and refreshes us. We can then operate more efficiently when we return once again to Beta. Just the act of sitting quietly listening to the sound of your breath, walking in the park, listening to music or just being quiet, can help the brain shift into Alpha. Alpha can be achieved readily when we go into a meditative state or start sensing things rather than thinking them. In addition, there are also the states of Theta and Delta brain waves that we attain in a deeper meditative state or when we are asleep.

Recognising Different Types of Intelligence

Intelligence is generally measured by how good children are at left brain processes such as mathematics. Society tends to reward and value this type of intelligence however there are many different types of intelligence. In his book *"Raising a Magical Child"* author, Joseph Chilton Pearce discusses the seven intelligences: Physical, Intellectual, Social, Emotional, Conceptual, Intuitive and Imaginative. While schools strive to educate children it tends to be restricted to left-brain processes and tends to ignore many elements within the child. Meditation helps children to develop a broad range of intelligences and is a simple way to help balance left and right brain learning. It is important that all aspects of a child's intelligence are recognised and nurtured. *Published by Dutton, New York, 1992.*

Meditation and Healing

There are many books written on the use of meditation (especially using visualisation and guided imagery) to help heal the body. As discussed earlier, visualisation can help to obtain desired goals by mentally rehearsing their achievement. Using meditation lowers stress and anxiety levels as well as managing pain and maintaining a positive outlook. These factors encourage the body to heal quickly. In medical research the placebo effect sheds some more light on this. During treatment trials and research, some patients report a beneficial effect following a treatment when in fact they have only received a placebo. This is because of positive expectations engendered which leads to a beneficial outcome rather than the use of drugs or interventions. The patient only "thinks" he or she has taken medicine, when in fact it is the confidence and positive outlook that has created the healing. The capacity of the mind, and its ability to aid in healing, is still unknown, however more researchers are looking into mind-body medicine and the link between emotions and disease.

There are several visualisations in this book that can be used for children who are injured or unwell which may help his or her condition. They are listed in the values/issue index at the back of the book.

Left and Right Brain

Meditation can help to synchronise the wave patterns in the left and right hemispheres of brain. This can help the brain to communicate more effectively and function with more clarity and focus. Researchers have found that children who display characteristics of ADHD or ADD are often more often right brain oriented. They learn through the creative, spatial, artistic and physical. They are very visual but also tactile learners. Our current school system is generally focused on the left-brain orientation. Generally teachers use blackboards and whiteboards and children are listening and watching the teacher in order to learn. Often right-brained children see and hear the information being taught but don't process it. They become distracted and this may lead to disruptive behaviour. It is interesting to note that some studies have found that right-brained learners, when given something in their hands to touch and sense, such as play-dough, tend to focus better in class.

Children with Learning Difficulties

Labelling children is always a challenging issue. Labels are used to describe and identify but they can be very restrictive. Sarah Wood discusses in her book *"Sensational Meditation for Children"*, that labelling people can restrict them to some degree because they tend to fulfil preconceived notions of "who we think they are". She goes on to discuss that we help the child most by creating the best possible learning environment without defining the behaviour. She adds that by avoiding labels children are then open to perceive themselves in a positive light. Meditation can help to provide a positive, calm learning environment.

Meditation has been used with great success with children diagnosed with ADHD, ADD, Asperger's Syndrome and Autism. Children described as "at risk" or having behavioural problems have also benefited from using meditation and calming techniques. Although anecdotal, there are significant positive results reported from teachers and parents whose pupils or children have participated in meditation.

Teachers whose students practice visualisation and guided imagery have observed significant improvements in concentration, listening skills, memory and focus. Many of the other improvements include a stronger sense of responsibility and discipline, ability to express feelings, ability to deal with conflict without negative physical actions, improved creative and abstract thinking, improved creative writing and artwork, being calmer, improved listening and a greater empathy for others.

If you take into account that many of the disorders list the following common symptoms or indicators;

- Difficulty focusing and concentrating
- Difficulty following instructions
- Irrational energy output or hyperactivity
- Difficulty listening
- Learning difficulties
- Tantrums/mood Swings

then it makes sense that learning meditation and calming techniques can only be of benefit. It will take time and plenty of practice and as discussed, is not an overnight cure all, however it provides parents with some alternatives and a guide to helping a child find the calm within them.

Types of Meditation

There are many different types of meditation that have originated from the diverse and rich cultures of the world. Meditation can be examined by way of the culture that produced it, the way it is practiced, the belief systems it is based on, how the person focuses their attention, as well as the motives and desire for meditation. Sometimes this examination can be very confusing to the first time meditator.

Although the names and types of meditation may vary, the common element is giving the mind, while in a calm and quiet state, something to focus on. Here are a few ways that Meditation is generally assessed:

- Following the Breath
- Connecting to the Body
- Walking/Movement Meditation
- Meditation on a sound or word (Mantra)
- Visualisation
- Mindfulness or meditation observing the mind
- Transcendental Meditation

There are many books listed in the resources section of this book that discuss all the different types of meditation and go into much greater detail. I also touch on some of the different types of meditation in the section on *Mini Meditations*.

Meditation with Children

For children's meditation I use a technique called Visualisation. It is my belief that we cannot teach children meditation in the same way we would use for adults. Techniques for children should predominantly help them to relax, teach them self-awareness and help them to believe in their potential. Visualisation can help children find a quiet safe place within their own mind and body.

As children mature they can try other meditative techniques or develop visualisation further. I also like to teach children some mindfulness practices. In addition to this I recommend adopting breath and body awareness activities and positive affirmations (positive self-talk) as a part of their meditation practice. Suggested affirmations are included with each visualisation in this book. It helps the parent or teacher to select an appropriate meditation, provides a positive outlook and enables the meditation to be focused. Some of the *Mini Meditations* briefly introduce other forms of classical meditation practice such as repeating a mantra (*in this case a positive affirmation),* focusing on an object and focusing on the breath. These activities are all written especially for children and are a great way to teach children how to relax.

What is Visualisation?

Simply put, visualisation is creating an image in the mind. A visualisation meditation involves being verbally guided, or mentally guiding yourself through a scene or scenario. Every person has the ability to visualise. In fact every time you think, your mind creates an image. Children think using images all the time. Sometimes these images come from a memory and sometimes they come from your imagination. Think of the one of your funniest times in your life and I am sure a smile will appear on your face as the images and feelings associated with this memory come into your mind. This is visualisation! Now imagine your ideal holiday destination or your dream-home -- this is visualising an event that has not yet occurred. Although you have not experienced these events physically, the feelings and images associated with your creative imagination have "lived" inside your mind.

Our mind is an amazing organ with incredible potential, most of which we are yet to understand. Olympic athletes and many other sport participants use visualisation to prepare for their events and as part of their training programs. Athletes picture themselves running faster, jumping higher or shooting the winning basket. Basically the mind doesn't differentiate between when you are actually performing your sport or whether you are rehearsing it in your mind through creative visualisation.

The visualisation process has also been used by people who are unwell or injured to aid in accelerating their recovery and healing their body. They imagine their body healing and getting better; they "see" themselves well and create positive mental pictures. Some of our greatest business leaders, scientists, artists and visionaries attribute much of their success to visualisation. This technique is a great tool to equip our children with.

Visualisation helps children to create positive thoughts and images which can prepare them for personal success and happiness. It can help to reprogram negative thoughts into positive ones. Visualisation teaches the child to concentrate on the image they are creating in their mind. This practice strengthens their ability to focus the mind during meditation, and when studying other subjects in the classroom.

Visualisation encourages creativity

Visualisation and the Imagination

"Imagination is more important than knowledge"- Albert Einstein

Our imagination is a powerful thing. If we can imagine a scenario, our body responds accordingly. Often our brain does not differentiate between what is real and imagined. If we imagine ourselves in a scenario that is calm and relaxed, such as sitting by the ocean listening to the waves, we will feel calm and relaxed and our body responds accordingly. Visualisation can help to obtain desired goals by mentally rehearsing the process of accomplishing them.

Although visualisation suggests that creating a mental image is only visual, it also involves imagining sounds, smell, feelings, touch and taste. The imagination responds to a variety of stimuli and we need to reinforce a child's natural ability to learn using all their sensory images. The visualisations in this book teach children to become aware of their body and to use breath awareness and affirmations to stimulate the imagination. The scenarios invite children to look, listen, taste, feel and smell and to use all areas of their imagination. They explore areas of personal development and key values as part of the meditation adventure, coupled with positive thinking, confidence, peace and tranquillity.

Instead of listening to a story passively, the child actually participates in the adventure and has the opportunity to experience it and picture it in their mind. Children can tap into their creativity and imagination to make the story their own and to see where the adventure takes them. Our imagination is not encouraged or stimulated much these days as most of it is done for us by the amazing media applications that technology has presented us with.

The visualisations and exercises in this book prepare children to be able to visualise on their own and take themselves through their own scenarios. Imagine a child visualising themselves calm and relaxed before an exam, or a child who can problem-solve by visualising the outcome. Imagine a child who takes a deep breath before responding to a negative situation by visualising themselves calm and with a positive outcome. A child who is having trouble making friends can visualise themselves happy and surrounded by friends. This makes children feel better and sets a positive expectation in their minds - in contrast to a child who looks sad and thinks he or she will never make any friends. Which child to you think will attract new friends?

Children who can tap into their imagination are more creative, better problem solvers and tend to perform better in school tasks because they learn more effectively.

If you can imagine it, you can achieve it.
If you see it, you can be it.

Is Visualisation Meditation?

Visualisation on its own is not actually meditation in the truest sense. However, when visualisation is practiced as a form of meditation, it is a great starting point for young children because they are very receptive to visualisation which can help them to develop the habit of attentive stillness in a fun and imaginative way. It also prepares the pathway for true meditation.

Often the words meditation and visualisation are used interchangeably. I like to look at the overall practice as meditation with visualisation being a technique that is used as part of the process. The breathing and body awareness activities or *warm-ups*, act as a way to release tension and any excess energy. The breathing, affirmations and beginning sequence help to focus a child's energy. This practice centres and relaxes them, ready for the visualisation. The visualisation is the stimulus that helps the child maintain focus and remain in this relaxed but mentally alert state. The ending sequence and *cool downs* gently bring the child out of the meditative state.

Guided Meditation

Guided meditation is a spoken meditation being offered by another person. This kind of meditation is an excellent way for a child to learn how to meditate as they are given imagery, symbols and prompts to follow on their journey. The imagery takes the visualisation process one step further by guiding the images towards a specific goal. The visualisations in this book have been written as guided meditations.

Being Mindful

Mindfulness Meditation is a type of meditation that requires us to be aware of our thoughts, feelings, emotions and other sensations in the present moment. This is another form of meditation that children respond well to and it can assist children to be calm and to deal with distractions and stressors. Children become more aware of what is within so they can deal with what is going on around them in a productive, less reactive way. The visualisations in this book help children to become aware of their thoughts, feelings and emotions. An excellent resource that explores this area further is "*The Mindful Child*" by Susan Kaiser Greenland.

Affirmations

Anyone who has read any of my books or used any of my products knows the value I place on using positive affirmations and positive thought. Teaching children to use affirmations and to focus on the positive things in their life encourages them to feel content and happy. It is such a simple and wonderful tool for children to embrace. We probably all remember the old saying of the half glass of milk. Positive people describe it as half full and negative will see it as being half empty. The half-full mindset will take children along a much happier and more successful pathway in life. Affirmations can assist the relaxation process, or when visualising and as part of general meditation practice.

Simply put, an affirmation is a statement of intention that you make to yourself and declare to be true. Repeating the affirmation strengthens its effect. In a typical day, we think and say many affirmations and have many thoughts both positive and negative. These thoughts and affirmations help to create our experiences.

Teaching children to repeat a positive statement helps them to believe that it is true in their subconscious mind. In essence we create what we think about. Therefore, if we teach children to use positive words and create positive thoughts it will evoke positive emotions. Positive emotions are stepping-stones that lead to positive expectations, which in turn lead to the creation of positive experiences. Think positive and you will attract positive. Think negative and you will attract negative. For example, say there are two children getting ready to attend school, one is saying over and over *I hate school and that school is boring*. The other child is saying, *I enjoy learning new things. Who* do you think will have the better day? The negative talk promotes the negative thoughts and will bring about negative experiences in the day because, in essence, that is what the child is expecting, either consciously or unconsciously. The child who has positive expectations will be in a much better frame of mind for the school day ahead. Positive expectations and a positive outlook will always positively affect the child's self-esteem. The latest research in this field also indicates that the body's biochemistry is also affected by our thought patterns.

Affirmations are a fantastic way to help children change negative thought patterns. Children pick up on these negativity patterns from adults around them just as they are affected by preconceived ideas that are often unintentionally placed in their growing minds. They pick up on statements such as, *He will never be very good at maths; no-one in our family has ever been able to draw; today is going to be a bad day; nothing ever goes right for us.* Then in their subconscious mind these negative thoughts become true for them. We start to believe what we hear.

During year ten high school I had chosen to take a special computing class. I was looking forward to the class and learning about this new technology. Unfortunately the teacher who took the class was a very surly and unfriendly gentleman who spent most of the class time telling us that we were hopeless and the worst class he had ever taught. Sadly, we believed him and I took an instant negative stance towards computers because I thought they were too difficult. I did not want to touch them and my little mantra of: "*I am no good with computers*" *became* a negative affirmation which manifested, of course! It was not until my early twenties that I had a mentor who helped me discover that I was not hopeless with computers and that in fact computers could be fun! My belief system changed in an instant because I had released all those negative thoughts I had built around computers. Now working with computers is a joyous activity.

Affirmations can help to change any way of thinking as well as old negative thought patterns. If we empower children with the knowledge that they can choose, monitor and change their own thoughts with the power of words, we can help them to create a peaceful life. With the thousands of thoughts we have everyday it is important for children to realise that some of them will be negative and instead of feeling guilty, to simply dismiss it and replace it with a positive thought. Older children can explore where the negative self-talk may have originated from and work on positive thoughts and words to help change or replace it.

When creating affirmations, they should always be positive and written or spoken in the present tense as if the statement is a statement of the current situation. For example good affirmations might be: *I am special. All my wishes comes true, I enjoy everything I do.* I suggest reading the affirmation out at the beginning of the meditation and again at the conclusion.

It is a personal choice whether to use affirmations or not with meditation. I find children enjoy them and it teaches them to use positive self-talk. Affirmations can be a powerful tool when used with visualisation as they make firm the images being created. If you are visualising relaxing on the beach and then repeating *I am calm, I am relaxed* -- the chances are you will be relaxed and calm as you are telling your subconscious mind that you are indeed calm!

Check out *The Affirmation Garden* picture book or CD for children at www.indigokidz.com.au

I am calm   I am kind to others

I am peaceful   I am powerful

I enjoy taking deep breaths

I have potential   I listen to others

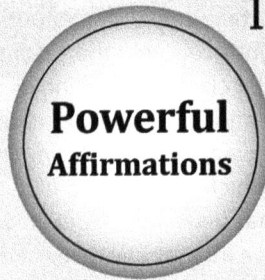

I can   **Powerful Affirmations**   I feel calm and relaxed

do it

I am unique

I believe in myself   I dream magical dreams

I treat others with respect

I enjoy being quiet and still

I have lots of wonderful friends

Hints for Writing Affirmations

▨ **Write in the present tense and say them as if they already exist**
Example*: I am Happy* **not** *I am going to be Happy.*

▨ **Make sure that they are always positive**
Example: *I feel fantastic* is a positive affirmation, *I feel miserable* is a negative affirmation.

▨ **State what you want, not what you don't want**
I feel safe and secure not *I am not scared.*

▨ **Write them so they are easy to understand**
Keep your affirmations short and simple so they are easy to say and remember. Make sure you write them in your own words. For a child the affirmation should reflect their age, vocabulary level and interests.

▨ **Believe what you are saying**
Make sure the affirmation feels right and is believable. Affirmations should evoke positive emotions and feelings. Combining affirmations with a visual image can help to reinforce the affirmation, especially for children.

▨ **Repeat them often**
Affirmations should be repeated as many times in a day as possible, especially when having a negative thought.

▨ **Use different ways to affirm**
Affirmations can be read quietly. You can write them, visualise them, say them in your mind, or read them out loud. You can sing affirmations, record them, cut out pictures that represent them or dance to them, whatever feels the most comfortable.

Some great ways to start affirmations

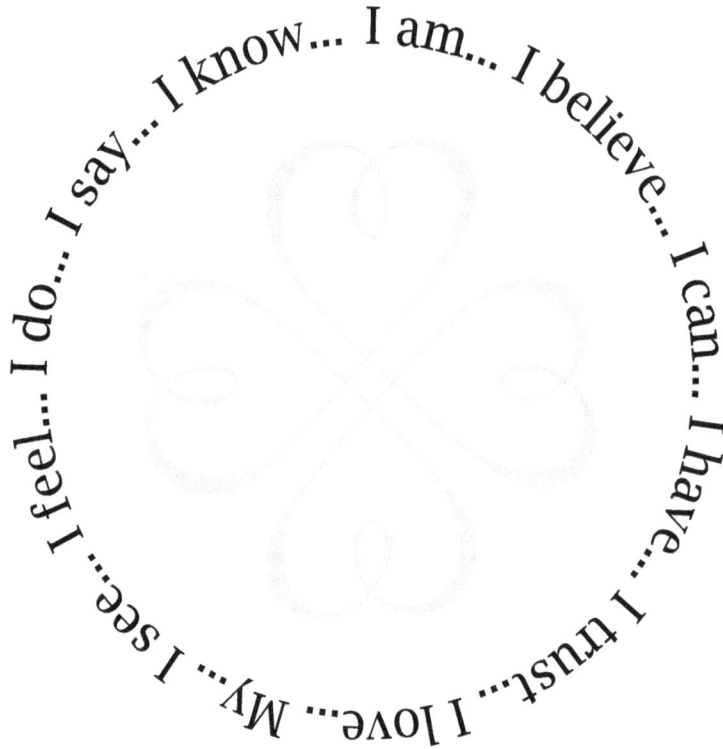

I know... I am... I believe... I can... I have... I trust... I love... My... I see... I feel... I do... I say...

Teaching Meditation and Relaxation to Children

Background and Getting Started

Here are some of the basics to teach meditation to children. It does not matter if you are doing a full meditation practice, a visualisation, a relaxation exercise or calming technique, the basic principles permeate across all practices.

What Makes a Good Meditation Teacher?

If you are teaching meditation to children, whether you are a parent or teacher, then it is a good idea to be a meditator yourself so you are teaching from a place of experience. When you participate in meditation for yourself you will know, by experience, the many benefits and some of the problems that can arise. Integrating meditation and relaxation techniques into your personal life assists you with managing your own stress levels and ensures that you are a calmer role model. As long as you are a relaxed, supportive and positive role-model this is a great start. By participating with your class or family you will become part of the experience and enjoy the benefits. There are some great meditation starter books available for adults. I have listed them in the reference section. I especially like *The Quiet* by Paul Wilson.

Where

Children need to meditate in a comfortable environment and can do this lying on the floor, sitting in a chair, sitting in a circle, in beanbags, with their heads on their school desks, lying on the grass or anywhere they feel safe, secure and comfortable. It also needs to be a practical space for a parent or teacher.

If meditating indoors, soft lighting helps to create the right atmosphere. The room should have no direct or strong sunlight beaming and be well ventilated. Make sure there is not too much clutter or mess around. Clothing should be comfortable and it is a good idea to loosen anything that is tight. Shoes should be removed. As children will be lying still they can sometimes get cold, so if practical, light blankets or soft cotton sheets can be used to keep them warm. These can be made relatively cheaply for a class and are easy to access at home.

To ensure that your child is comfortable and not wriggling around it is a good idea to help him or her to find their comfortable position beforehand. Make sure they are not touching anyone else and have plenty of room around them. There is more information specific to the setting in the chapters on *Teaching Meditation at Home* and *Teaching Meditation in Schools*.

When

Meditation can be done at anytime. Many experienced meditators like to start and finish their day with meditation but this is not always practical for parents and teachers. For parents/caregivers I would suggest doing meditation at night time in bed and allowing the child to drift off in to a peaceful sleep or as part of a relaxing night time routine. If your child is upset, angry or out of sorts then this is also a good time to meditate together. For teachers, first thing in the morning or immediately after lunch is a good time. This time refreshes the children and is good preparation for the day or afternoon ahead. Meditating at a similar time each day is beneficial as it helps with the preparation for meditation and making it part of a regular routine.

Posture

If sitting, children should be encouraged to sit cross-legged with a straight spine and shoulders back. Explain to them that a straight spine with help with their breathing and the energy flow throughout the body. If sitting on the floor, then use a high cushion or folded blanket under the buttocks to help keep the hips higher than the knees as this may be more comfortable. If children find sitting cross-legged too uncomfortable they can try sitting with their back against a wall. If sitting in a chair then a small cushion can be placed in the small of the back to aid support, but make sure feet are flat on the floor. Hands can be comfortably placed in laps, or on knees with palms upward. Another popular position for the hands is for the thumb and first finger to be joined on both hands with palms upward, resting on the knees.

As children develop their meditation practice they may want to try some different hand positions or poses known as *Mudras. Mudras* are said to help in the meditation process by focusing the body as well as the mind. With younger children in a home situation you may like to have them sitting on your lap so you can gently rub the back or their arm or leg in a soft repetitive motion. This is very soothing and helps to settle them.

If children are lying down on the floor then a straight spine is still important. Encourage children when possible to lie flat on their back with their arms by their sides and to have their hands with palms facing up. If a child regularly falls asleep during meditation you may suggest that they try sitting up. Interestingly, many teachers report that they are sure that some of the children are asleep during the meditation, because they appear still and their breathing is so relaxed and rhythmic. However as soon as they say it is time to wriggle the fingers and toes, the children respond immediately. This indicates that they have not been asleep but in a state of active relaxation.

Encourage your child or children to close their eyes for the meditation. This helps with distractions and the process of visualising. Some children may need to place their hands over the eyes to begin with or you can use eye pillows (see *Meditation Aids on Page 60*). Some children may simply want to look down at the floor or close their eyes half-way. If children are fearful of closing their eyes then I suggest letting them keep their eyes open.

Basic Meditation Posture

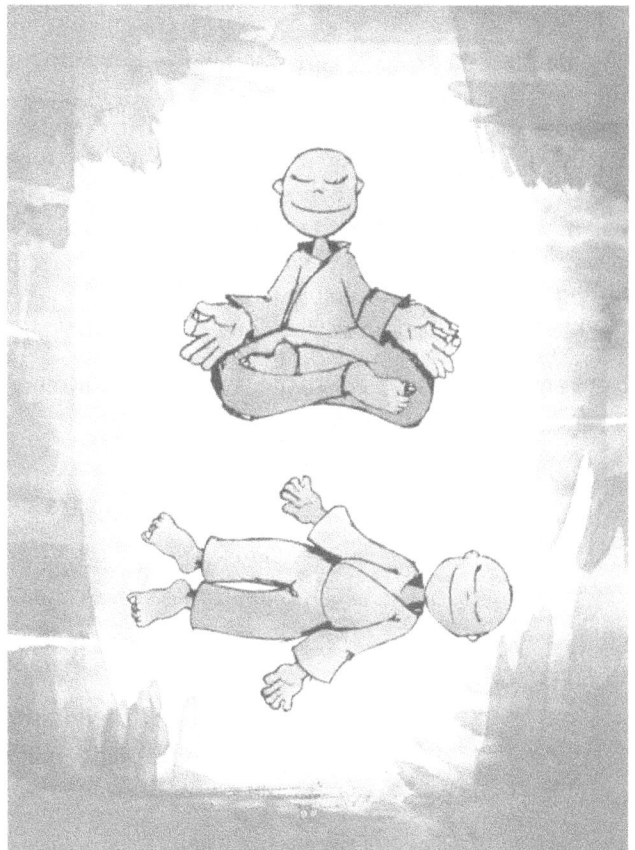

Mudras

Mudra (pronounced moo-dra) is another of these terms that can have a myriad of definitions. Generally a Mudra refers to unique hand gestures and finger postures used in meditation practice. These postures or gestures help to focus and guide energy flow and reflexes to the brain. They are often referred to as a type of hand therapy and can be done with one hand or both hands.

Mudra's can be seen as a form of non-verbal communication and mode of self-expression. Mudras are used throughout the world by many different cultures and religions. Some cultures believe that each of our five fingers represents one of the five elements. The thumb is fire, forefinger is air, the middle finger is ether, the ring finger is earth and the little finger is water. Keeping these five elements balanced will lead to optimal health. Each Mudra is said to have its own particular effect.

Like meditation, Mudras can be practiced anywhere, anytime. You can practice a Mudra whilst sitting, lying or standing. You can even practice when walking. Mudras have been said to help with synchronising left and right brain functioning, health issues, improved concentration, memory and creativity. Mudras can be done on their own with some deep breathing or as a support for meditation. I always reinforce with children that they are a great relaxation tool that can be done when they are upset or worried, bored, feeling spacey or unwell and are great to do when travelling. Children can have fun making up their own.

I do not pretend to be an expert on Mudras but from my experience these are the ones I find most beneficial to use with children. You may wish to explore others and will find that there are slightly different spellings, methods of practice and effects based on their origins. I use simple terms that children can relate to when discussing Mudras. I explain that Mudras are great exercise for the hands. It is like yoga for the hands. Practicing Mudras can help them to concentrate while meditating. I discuss that Mudras also help you to feel calm and balanced. I always practice the different Mudras with children and let them pick what like the best or feel most comfortable with. Children love trying the different Mudras and will often pick a favourite one that they use during meditation. You can discuss how each one makes them feel and some of the associated properties of the Mudras. Mudras can also be done with the whole body.

Here are some basic Mudra's that I use with children. All of these Mudras involve using both hands. I have given them modified names suitable to children.

Balance Mudra

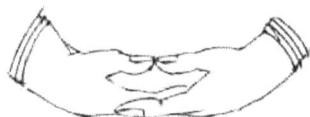

This Mudra is one of the most commonly used during meditation and is also known as the Dyhani or Dhyana Mudra. It is sometimes called the Yoga Mudra. It is a classical meditation pose depicting contemplation and connection with universe. It helps to create calm and balance.

Relax both hands in your lap as if making a bowl with the left hand lying on top of the right hand and the thumbs gently touching each other.

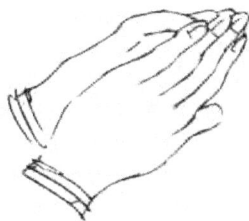

Prayer Mudra

This Mudra is also commonly used and supports harmony and peace. It is very good for balancing the left and right brain and centering. It helps with listening and focusing. It is also a pose of silence. It can also be called the Namaste or Namaskara Mudra. It is a good pose to use to start your meditation session before moving onto a different Mudra. Please note young children may not be able to hold this pose for very long.

Place both hands gently pressing together and facing upwards at the centre of the chest around the height of the heart.

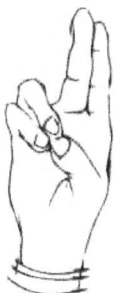

Health Mudra

This Mudra is good for the immune system, illness, infections and to support vision. It helps to reduce fatigue and is good for self-confidence. This is also known as the pran, prana or Life Mudra.

With each hand, fold the little finger and the ring finger to the thumb to form a circle. Extend the remaining fingers.

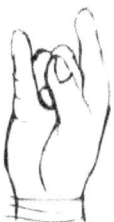

Energy Mudra

This Mudra is good for balancing energy and helps to detoxify the body (Also known as the Apan Mudra).

With each hand place the middle finger and ring finger together on the thumb. Extend the other fingers upward. When meditating in a sitting position hands normally rest on the outer leg towards the knee with palms facing up. When lying, arms rest gently by the side with palms facing up.

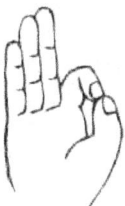

Wisdom Mudra

Also known as the Gyan, Guyan or Gyana Mudra. This Mudra helps grounding and calms and clears the mind. It also promotes a peaceful night's sleep and is said to promote wisdom and improve concentration.

With each hand place the tip of the thumb and the index finger together. Extend the remaining three fingers in a relaxed and joined position.

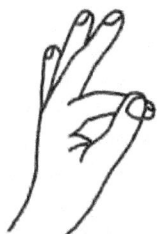

Confidence Mudra

Also know as the Ahkamkara Mudra. This Mudra is good to boost self-confidence and to help with being more assertive. It helps to counteract fear.

With each hand bend the index fingers slightly and put the upper joint of the thumb to the side of the middle joint of the index finger. Extend the remaining fingers.

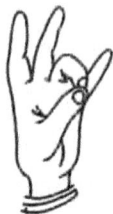

Earth Mudra

This Mudra is good for grounding when you are feeling scattered or unsettled. This Mudra can help you feel strong and secure and re-assured.

With each hand, place the tips of the ring finger and the thumb together. Extend the remaining fingers.

How Often?

With young children it is dependant on a few variables. At home you may do a meditation every night as part of their bedtime routine or have regular nights put aside. In a class situation teachers may offer it each day for 10-15 minutes to start the day or after lunch. It may be a special activity that is done once a week or as needed. The more regularly it is performed, the more beneficial it is to the child and it becomes part of life rather than being a quick fix. There is more information in the chapters *Teaching Meditation at Home* and *Teaching Meditation in Schools.*

Tone of Voice

When reading the visualisation, use a soft, slow voice. I often lower my voice and find this has a more soothing quality. Give the child a chance to visualise the scene and pause where necessary. You can observe the children meditating and decide whether to speed up or slow down the meditation. Try not to walk around the room as this can be distracting for young children as they try to follow your voice.

Music

You can play soft background music or have complete silence. I find that relaxing music (with no words), softly playing in the background helps to relax children and to set the scene for the meditation. Music is calming and helps the child tune out any other distracting noises. This is particularly helpful in a class situation as noise from other classrooms or the playground can be very distracting for beginners. As children develop with their meditation skills they will be able to use the sounds around them as part of their routine and learn to acknowledge them then move on in their meditation practice. Complete silence works just as well. It is up to the individual teacher or parent.

Meditation Aids

There are many meditation aids but I like a simple practical approach with children otherwise the focus becomes on "things" rather than the practice of meditation itself.

As discussed previously, pillows and blankets can be useful for children if you have access to them. If children are lying on the floor they often like to have a blanket over them for warmth and security or they may lie on top of them. Pillows or cushions can be used for sitting on and to help support the hips and spine. Eye pillows can also be used to help children with keeping their eyes closed and to minimise distractions.

Wendy, a very resourceful year one teacher I met at a yoga course, had her mother in law sew up linseed eye pillows for her class. The linseed and material for the eye pillows cost approximately $20.00 for the whole class. The eye pillows were made from a piece of silky material and each one needed around 20cm x 30cm.

Three kilograms of flaxseed was needed for 24 bags, each bag had approximately 125gms of flaxseed in them. Flaxseed is available in bulk at grocery shops. A parent who worked for a furniture company donated some material. The heavier material was made into mini mats for the children to lie down on and the lighter material was made into mini blankets, to go over the children.

Wendy has also made pillows up for children in Pre-Primary. At the beginning of the year, they design and then draw their design onto their pillow with fabric crayons. It is then ironed by an adult. The children then stuff and sew up the pillows themselves. This activity encompasses the learning areas of Technology, Maths and Art.

Starting Age

There is no set age to start children meditating. I have found a good age to start preparing for meditation is about four or five years of age, however it depends on a child's development and their attention span. You will be able to tell if your child is ready. My daughter started the process of learning to meditate at the age of four and I have seen great success with kindergarten-aged children. With younger children just asking them to close their eyes and practice some deep breathing while listening to a story is a good start. They can begin listen to the words and imagine the characters or scenes. This is a great way to prepare for meditation and to encourage their interest. You can adjust the language used in the visualisations or activities or modify the visualisations to suit the child's age. Many of the activities in the section on *Relaxation and Calming Techniques* can be used or modified for very young children.

Time

The visualisations in this book vary in length. Most of them will take between five and 15 minutes. Each visualisation is left with an open-ended invitation to continue the adventure. The time children are actually meditating can vary from seconds to minutes. This will increase with practice.

I like to complete the last sentence of the visualisation i.e. "*Stay as long as you like relaxing in your bubble bath enjoying the warmth*" and then let the child stay in the meditation. You may need to say: "*I am going to be very quiet now and let you continue to relax or continue your adventure.*" The child will get used to this quiet time at the end of the meditation session. It gives the child a chance to further explore their imagination and be creative.

It is up to the individual parent or teacher to decide how long to keep the child in the meditation. Follow your instincts and you will know the child's attention span. When reading the visualisation use the prompts and paragraph breaks to allow the children time to visualise. The visualisations are open ended so that you can allow your child or class time at the end to stay in the visualisation. You may start with 30 seconds and build up to a few minutes. You can then conclude the meditation.

Learning with all Senses

The visualisations often ask the child an open-ended question such as *What can you see?* It is important to emphasise that not every child will see a clear picture and this is perfectly normal. During meditation some children will feel or use their sense of touch (kinaesthetic), some will see a mental image i.e. pictures, colours or symbols (visual) and some will learn from the words or sounds (auditory). Some children will associate a taste or smell or in the case of kinaesthetic learners they may actually feel how their body responds to things either emotionally or through movement. It is important to remember that children not only sense in a variety of ways but they also learn in a variety of ways.

Each child's experience will be different based on how they learn and process information. The visualisations in the book incorporate all three learning styles and prompt all of the senses so that the child can experience meditation in a way that suits. For example, *What can you see? Does it feel smooth or rough? What do you hear? How does it make you feel? What can you smell?* I have observed children drawing or moving their hands during meditation, sometimes you can see them smiling or nodding their heads in response. It is important to encourage all types of natural learning abilities.

Note: There is a special visualisation *The Magic Factory* that has been written to make children aware of all their senses and suggests left and right images to both sides of the brain. This is an excellent one for discussion afterwards.

Choosing a Visualisation

You can randomly select a visualisation or work your way through the book. You may wish to choose your visualisation according to the affirmation or theme associated with it. This enables the parent or teacher to deal with issues that may be affecting the child or class. It is a good idea to read it beforehand so that you are comfortable with it. Feel free to use your own words and to use language to suit the age of your child or class. These visualisations are a guide only, an indication of what you can do. Explore the visualisations further if you wish. You may like to add your own ideas and adventures or make up a visualisation especially based on your child's needs or interests.

Affirmations

As discussed affirmations can be a powerful tool when used with visualisation as they reinforce the images and feelings that are being created. At the beginning of meditation practice I ask the children to repeat the affirmation 3-5 times to set the focus for the meditation, the affirmation can be said on the out breath, for example, Breathe in and on the out breath say *I am calm.* The affirmation helps to focus the mind of the reader as well as set the tone for the child. They can then repeat the affirmation at the end of the meditation.

Rainbow Thoughts

In addition to an affirmation, each visualisation in this book has rainbow thoughts associated with it. The rainbow thoughts provide teachers and parents with an insight to the key values and issues addressed in the visualisation. They also provide a focus or prompt for discussion or a sharing circle afterwards.

Boys and Girls

Rainbow Dreaming contains a mixture of masculine and feminine visualisations. The visualisations have been designed to allow children to experience balance and develop empathetic qualities. It is important to remind children that they are entering a world of imagination and fun and that anyone can be anything, there is no right or wrong. The characters in the visualisations are referred to as *he* or *she* alternately throughout the book.

Progressive Muscle Relaxation

Progressive muscle relaxation is a technique that involves progressively tensing then relaxing the muscles. When we are stressed our muscles naturally tense up. By creating then releasing muscle tension we are learning how to relax the tension in our muscles. Several of the visualisations and exercises in this book teach children how to do progressive muscle relaxation. It works very well with children who are having trouble getting to sleep.

Children that Won't

For meditation to be successful, the child must participate voluntarily. If they do not wish to participate don't force them. If children enjoy what they are learning then their interest will build and they will want to participate. Finding stillness will come the more they participate. As a parent or teacher this is very rewarding to see. You will know their limits and concentration spans. Teachers may find they have some children who have poor concentration. I would suggest putting them closest to you so that you can help to settle them if need be. It may also help to discuss with students that if they do not wish to participate they can lie quietly and rest while the class does their meditation or relaxation activity. More often than not they begin to feel more comfortable with the procedure and then join in later.

Beginning the Meditation

After reading the affirmation out loud, you may like to start each meditation with a special beginning routine that allows the child to start to focus and relax. Children like routines and I have found that the familiarity of the beginning sequence enables them to easily prepare for the meditation. The sequence teaches them to become aware of their breath to start with and to listen to the sound of their breathing.

Children are then taught to cover themselves in the white light of a moonbeam, let all their worries go with the Magic Worry Hat and then to put a special pendant around their neck to protect them. The moonbeam provides a focal point for the child and helps them to relax. The Moonbeam helps prepare the children and is a prompt for centering and starting the process of reaching a meditative state. How long a child is actually in a true meditative state during the visualisation will vary from child to child. The important thing is that they are working towards it and are learning the processes as part of the journey.

The "Worry Hat" helps children to clear their mind of any thought that is troubling them. We don't always know what upsets children and this gives them a chance to be in control of their worries and to let them go. The pendant provides a symbol of protection and helps the child to feel safe through their journey. The three important elements to remember are a cue to relax and focus, an opportunity to let go of their worries and to reinforce that they are safe.

There are three opening meditations for you to use. One is the full version that you may need until the child is used to it, then you can use the shortened version. There is also a slightly different alternative sequence for older children or those children who are more experienced. If you are feeling very creative you can make up your own beginning sequence. Children can ride a magic carpet, journey on a spaceship or open the gate to a garden or any other scenario because the possibilities are endless. You can use a worry tree, a worry bag or a worry pond instead of a hat. You can us a special person or animal friend to keep them company instead of the pendant.

It is a good idea to begin in the same way each time, especially for beginners, so they identify it as part of their relaxing and focusing routine. Have you noticed how every fairy story begins with; *Once upon a time*.

If you do not wish to use the beginning sequence simply start with some deep breaths and *Imagine...*

Pausing the Meditation

Each visualisation provides an opportunity for children to continue the meditation for a period of time without being verbally guided. Paragraph breaks indicate a place where you may like to pause to allow the child time to visualise and process. It is also good to pause for a few moments after a question is posed in the script i.e. Can you hear the sound of the birds? or when there is a spoken part in italics such as *I am calm I am calm*. This allows time to visualise and process what they have been asked or prompted to do.

In each visualisation you will come to the words: *Spend as long as you like ...* This is the cue to leave children for a few minutes to participate in the visualisation and to explore it further. You can then move on to conclude the meditation with your ending sequence. With beginners I suggest only leaving them for 30 seconds before moving on to the ending sequence and then gradually add more time as they get more competent. You will be able to judge from your child's or the class's reaction.

Ending the Meditation

Once you have decided to conclude the meditation, you can read the ending sequence. You may wish to put it into your own words. I then read the affirmation again to conclude the meditation.

The ending enables the child to return to the starting point of the meditation, in a logical sequence. They step back onto their moonbeam, hang up their pendant, walk past their Worry Hat (remind them that their worries stay in the hat and dissolve away) and back to where they started. Wriggling their fingers and toes helps to ground children.

If you do not wish to use the ending sequence then an alternative ending is suggested or simply finish with the open ended sentence and the affirmation.

At night time parents may want their child to drift off into a peaceful sleep at the open ended point of the meditation. This is up to the individual and a valid way to end the meditation.

The Beginning and Ending Sequences are located on Page 125

Meditation with Children for the First Time

Before starting meditation for the first time it is a good idea to run through some of the following activities with your child or class.

Introduce the Term Meditation

Discuss the word meditation and what it means. Include any terms you would like the child to be aware of, such as affirmation or inner vision. Children like to know why they are doing things, we all do. I often use the comparison that meditation is like exercise for the mind and I discuss some of the benefits with them. Appeal to the child's interests. If they are interested in sport, discuss how meditation can help. If they are artistic then you might want to talk about how meditation can increase their creativity. I also discuss how meditation helps us to expand our levels of awareness helping us experience and notice what is going on around us and how this affects other people.

Make sure you use simple, practical language and explanations. Remember that children seem to understand that meditation helps us to listen to our heart's messages. This helps us to understand our thoughts and feelings and that leads us to feeling happier and more content.

We might use examples to illustrate these points and include likening the mind to a dirty muddy pond where you can't see the bottom. Meditation helps cleanse away the mud and debris making the pond clear so we can see everything again. The process of visualisation can be described as listening to a special kind a story but instead of just hearing the word, they will create and draw the story in their minds. They will have the opportunity to experience and explore this story and they will feel great afterwards.

Give the children a chance to ask questions and discuss their own definitions.

Inner Vision

The concept of seeing pictures in the mind is easy to teach children and a great starting point for meditation.

- Ask the child to close their eyes and picture what their favourite toy/possession looks like
- Discuss how they saw the object if their eyes were closed
- Explain to them that this is inner vision or seeing a picture in your mind or head

You can ask children to imagine that there is a special place in their head, between their eyes and on top of their nose that is like a special picture screen. When you use your imagination and visualise, this is where the pictures appear. This can be described as their inner vision or inner eyes.

You can practice with other objects from their bedroom or classroom. You can then progress to picturing a whole room, or their home. Simple things such as fruit, vegetables, their pets and family members also work well for those beginning meditation.

Mind Talk

During the meditations, the child often has to repeat an affirmation or phrase in their mind. As discussed above in the section on Inner Vision, the meditations may ask them an open ended question such as, *What can you see*? At home it may not matter if they repeat it out loud but in a group/class situation it can be distracting. You can try the following activity.

- Ask the child to say their name out loud
- Now ask them to say it without speaking
- Explain, this is talking in the quiet of your mind, that you don't need to say the words out loud because your mind can still hear them

Try other examples to ensure they have understood the concept. Ask them to sing a favourite nursery rhyme or repeat a popular saying. Explain that during the meditation the questions are given to encourage them to think about quietly or answer in their mind. One teacher who works with pre-primary students explains to the children that they have an inner mouth as well as inner eyes and children enjoy this concept. If a child has difficulty talking in the quiet of their mind, then ask them to talk in a very soft whisper or mouth their answer just with their lips without speaking.

Meditation Manners

When learning to meditate I like to encourage children to learn some "meditation manners," especially in a class situation. I don't like to think of them as rules, the fewer restrictions the better. Some of these have been discussed in this chapter previously but I will touch on them again. You may like to adapt them to suit your family or class. Here are some that I like to talk about with children.

* Everyone has a right to meditate or participate in relaxation time
* Respect your class or family member's right to participate. If you do not wish to participate then you must not distract others (talking, giggling, touching)
* When meditating you need to find a comfortable position and your own space. Respect other's space and do not touch others
* When participating in discussions or doing a follow up activity, remind children that anyone can be anything in these meditations and if they do not wish to discuss their meditation then that is their choice. There is no right or wrong. Everyone's ideas are important and valid. We may not all experience the same things and this is perfectly okay. Meditation is not a competition but something we can all enjoy in our own unique way.

Comfortable Position

As discussed earlier in the book it is a good idea to let beginners experiment until they find their comfortable position. You can discuss the various postures and positions and let them practice each one. Remember what is comfortable to them may not look that comfortable to you as an adult.

Symbols

It is good to explain to a beginner that during meditation people may see symbols. Symbols can have a special meaning or significance. This symbol can be an object, picture, person, character or even a colour or sound that represents a certain concept. For example a child may see their pet dog during meditation, this may symbolise that they are safe and loved. My daughter always sees dolphins. I have had children say they have seen the colour green when they are not feeling well (green is a healing colour) and one child heard singing. You can discuss some of symbols that are used in everyday life i.e. a swimmer with a line through is a no swimming zone or the colour red symbolises **Stop** and is used on stop signs.

After the meditation children can share their experiences and if they have seen a symbol they may wish to draw it. A meditation journal is a good idea, as students can notice if certain patterns and symbols reoccur, either in meditation or during dreams or daydreams.

Moonbeam, Worry Hat and Crystal Pendant

Before meditating for the first time it is important to make children familiar with the symbols, objects or prompts you are going to use. In this case we are using the Moonbeam, the Magic Worry Hat and the Crystal

Pendant symbols. Discuss what a moonbeam may look like and perhaps do a mini-visualisation on being covered in warm white light. I always tell them that a moonbeam is magically strong and that they will never fall through it. It is like a special road and that they can walk or run anywhere they want on it.

Discuss how magical the Worry Hat is. I tell the children that the Magic Worry Hat dissolves all worries and busy feelings and is fresh and ready for them to wear again next time they do a meditation. It can take millions of worries away and is as vast as the universe. They can give the Magic Worry Hat as many worries as they want because there is no limit! There is an Activity on Page 261 that discusses making a Magic Worry Hat at home or for the class. Children can write down their worries and place them in the hat.

The crystal pendant is for protection and to make them feel safe. Discuss what their pendant looks like. They may like to draw it or make one so that it is easier to visualise. Of course if you have chosen other symbols, objects or prompts then discuss them.

Beginners' Problems

There are four main problem areas that sometimes arise. These problems occur with the most experienced meditators as well!

Problem Visualising
When this happens, explain that we can all do it even if we think we can't. Ask them if they have had any dreams at night and if they can remember them. Explain that dreams happen when we are asleep with our eyes closed yet we still see the pictures, so we can all visualise! We even visualise during our day dreams.

Picture in their Mind Fading
Some children have trouble keeping the picture they are seeing in their mind, they may report that it fades out. Tell them not to worry and not to try too hard to keep the image in their mind if it is slipping away. They can continue on in the meditation and try to bring the image back gently. This is something that will improve with practice.

Distracting Thoughts
Focus is one of the key aspects to meditation. You may find children have trouble concentrating or they may say to you that they started thinking about other things and their mind seemed to wander. This is a natural part of learning how to meditate. Even the most experienced meditators have straying attention and unrelated thoughts popping into their heads. Encourage them and let them know this is a normal part of the process. When this happens they can focus back on their breathing, and when ready, return to the words of the visualisation being spoken. With practice their attention will wander less and less. Concentration cannot be forced or children will be fighting against the very thing they are striving for.

Distractions
It takes some children quite a bit of time to get used to the process of being still. They may wriggle or get uncomfortable or say their legs hurt and dozens of other excuses. Noises outside may also distract them. It is all part of the learning process and again is something that will improve with practice. Try to remove major distractions from the home or classroom prior to meditation. Such things as mobile phones being switched off and a clear uncluttered space helps prepare the children for their meditation practice.

Some children who fidget may find the process easier if they are given a stress ball or ball of play dough or plasticine (or something similar) to hold in their hands and squeeze. Kinaesthetic learners respond especially well to this.

Important Points

- Remind children that once they have experienced any of the visualisations in the book, they can go back any time they need to. At times of stress or worry they can feel safe and calm by revisiting that special place in their mind for example, the garden in *The Magic Garden* or *The Quiet Cave.*
- Remember not to set your expectations too high and think that you will have your children sitting or lying perfectly still, this is not the objective - the process of meditating is. Like any new skill, meditation may take some time for children to learn and to be comfortable with. Continue giving positive reinforcement and encouragement and don't give up. Meditation should not be a form of forced concentration, it should occur in a relaxed state. Make sure you never show impatience. A calm, patient teacher or parent is great role-model.
- Keep your language and instructions simple.
- Don't have any preconceived ideas about how and when children will respond. Trust that meditation is of benefit and enjoy the process.
- Different emotions can arise during meditation. Children are very in tune and may see or experience things that we sometimes don't expect. These occasions are quite rare. Stories, smells, songs or pictures can trigger emotions and memories that are upsetting to a child. If a child is upset following a meditation let them know that these sad feelings will soon pass. Handle the child the way you would handle any other classroom or home situation where a child is upset. Be patient, kind and understanding and listen to the child, reassuring them. These emotions often help a child to learn a little more about themselves and may provide a valuable insight to the parent or teacher.
- Keep control of discussions, especially in a class situation. Children when learning to discuss meditations sometimes try to embellish or copy others. This is a natural part of the learning process. Gently guide them to their conclusion and keep reinforcing that they will all see or experience different things. There is no right or wrong. Don't be drawn into the details of the meditation and simply focus more on the process. Use questions such as, How did you feel? Were you able to concentrate today? Listening and being non-judgmental are crucial to this process.
- Remind children that they are safe at all times. Remind the children that they have their crystal pendant of protection with them at all times.
- You might get some giggling and wriggling at first. Children may talk and be restless. Just go with the flow, keeping relaxed and calm. There will always be distractions and at the end of the day children are much more adaptable and what may be a distraction to you is not to them.
- It may take one session, a few weeks or a school term to see the positive results, but they will come.
- There are no deep focusing meditations in this book. I find that these are more suited to children after puberty or adults.
- Try the exercises yourself and read the meditations before you do them with your children. You will see how they work and feel much more confident.
- Remember you can do the visualisations as part of a full meditation practice or use them on their own.

Teaching Meditation and Relaxation at Home

Creating a Calm Home

With our fast paced, noisy, time obsessed culture, home is often our only sanctuary. I have so many comments from people saying that when they enter our home they feel calm and relaxed and that it has a really good vibe. Anyone can achieve this feeling. Whether you rent, own an apartment, house, villa or caravan or even a holiday spot, there are lots of ways to create a calm home and help to create a holistic approach for our children. Here a few ideas that may help you to create a calm home that will help to nourish a child's soul and develop their spirit. Take what you want from this section. Some ideas will resonate with you and some won't. Just follow your instincts and feelings.

Walk the Walk

We cannot expect our kids to be calm if we are not calm ourselves. Our stress levels impact our kids, and to put it simply, stressed out parents equal stressed out kids. We are the role models they watch and learn from. Our behaviours, habits and reactions are a guide for them. In a world where we worry about children's overscheduled lives, perhaps it is actually the parents who are the most stressed, trying to meet home requirements, work commitments and their children's activities. If we simplify life we make things easier for everyone. Take time to meditate, even if it is just taking five minutes every day to do some deep breathing. Don't overload yourself or your family. If your kids have after-school activities and commitments try not to put yourself under too much pressure to get them there on time.

Take Care of Yourself

Parents are busy too and need some time out. Take some time to nurture yourself with a regular massage or body treatment or even a walk on the beach. Try a warm bath, yoga or some daily exercise to help you unwind. Getting a good night's sleep is very important so if you have trouble sleeping, try some of the calming strategies in this book. I like to have an essential oil bubble bath every Friday night. It is my routine and I look forward to this treat at the end of each week. I light candles, put some music on and totally relax. Find 10 minutes a day to meditate. First thing in the morning or just before bed is a good time. If you get into a routine it is much easier.

Work out a set of daily affirmations just for you and repeat them throughout the day. Try finding the time to stop each hour and take five deep breaths. Cut down on tea and coffee and drink plenty of water throughout the day. Remember, you can't keep taking care of others if you are not taking care of yourself-something will give.

Declutter and Organise

I am a firm believer in clutter-free homes. Clutter equals stress! Many books point to the benefits of de-cluttering and that an organised home is more peaceful and easier to maintain. My friends and family laugh that I have a label and basket for everything in the house but I find it so much easier to spend some initial time organising everything and then things are easy to find and put away. Thank goodness for those IKEA organiser sets, they are brilliant! I also find it is easier to keep the house clean, saving time and stress levels in the long run. Whilst our home is not minimalist-it is definitely uncluttered but still a warm family home. We have sold or given away over half the contents of our last house. We also regularly go through cupboards and remove things we have not used in the past six months. I start with three bags or boxes labelled: sell, donate and trash.

Do a shelf every night or a room once a week, but slowly work your way through your home, room by room. A de-cluttered home equals a de-cluttered mind! The energy flow is better. You will have more time and energy to spend with your family.

There are some great books and blogs on the topic of de-cluttering and minimalism filled with great ideas. The whole process is physically, mentally and spiritually liberating because it reinforces to everyone that "stuff" doesn't make you happy. See the resources section at the end of the book for more information.

Embrace the beauty of less and be content with what you have. Possessions don't make you happy!

Give your Children Time to Be

Children need time to be children. Try not to over structure your child's time. Make sure there is flexible, non-structured time during the week and on the weekends to just be. Teach your children to enjoy quiet time to simply read or relax. Encourage them to explore, create and simply be a kid having fun.

Colour

Colour is energy. Each colour has its own vibration and wavelength frequency and it can affect how we think and feel. Colour can change moods, evoke feelings and emotions and can even affect our behaviour. There have been many books written on the properties of colours and how people respond to them. Marketing Companies and Advertising Agencies are very aware of this and tap into it when doing such things as creating logos and developing branding. Think of all the colours used in children's toys and in children's television shows. Fast food chains and children's food products use bright colours to attract their customers. The brighter, more vibrant colours tend to stimulate and rejuvenate while softer, pale colours tend to relax. Great colours for relaxation are soft green, blue, violet, mauve, pink and cream. Please don't panic and repaint your house. This is a guide only and you can create a relaxing space using other suggestions in this book.

Peaceful Bedtime

Each family has its own way of handling bedtime and it can be tricky, especially when there is home work and other commitments to be considered. Most families will have their own bedtime routine. Personally, I like my children's bedrooms to be relaxing and peaceful. It should be a place for them to spend quiet time and relax in their own special space. If children's rooms are painted in calming colours this also helps. I try to keep them clutter free so they have a nice personal space. I suggest keeping televisions and computers in a separate area and keeping electrical appliances to a minimum, perhaps just a light and music player. Dedicate a special place in your office or a cupboard where all electronics "go to bed" during the night. In our home we encourage our children not to use any computer or electronic equipment within an hour of bedtime. We try and do stories, reading or drawing close to bedtime as it seems to have a relaxing affect. I often have lavender oil or a special harmony blend burning throughout the house at bedtime as I find this also has a calming effect.

It is important that children get a good night's sleep and it helps to have a set time to go to bed and a routine. Recent research estimates that up to 20% of children do not get a good night's sleep and irregular bedtimes can affect their learning potential. Sleep gives a young child's brain a chance to process what they have done in the day. Some studies show that currently our children sleep, on average, an hour less than they did 30 years ago. Reasons suggested for this include television, computer games and electronic devices, increased homework, extra curricular activities and parents home late from work wanting to spend more time with their children before bed.

Tips for a Peaceful Bedtime

- Set a time for bedtime
- Make bedtime part of a nightly routine i.e. have a bath or shower, brush teeth then quiet time
- Don't let children eat too close to bedtime
- Cut down stimulating activities about an hour prior to bedtime i.e. computer, television, electronic devices and video games
- Quiet time prior to bed can be fun, read stories together, play puzzles, have a cuddle, do some stretching or relaxation exercises
- For older children who have homework, make sure they have some quiet time before going to bed otherwise their mind will still be on their work and they will not sleep as well
- Play a relaxing meditation CD or music
- Meditate together or do a calming visualisation
- Make a bedtime atmosphere in the room i.e. soft lights, aromatherapy oils and soft calming music playing in the background. For younger children, have the child's favourite comforter with them i.e. favourite doll, rug, pillow, teddy or keepsake. Salt lamps make a great night lamp and are great for a relaxing bedroom atmosphere
- Say some bedtime affirmations together or make a special one that you say each night such as; *I can feel my body relaxing with each breath, I am calm and peaceful, I sleep peacefully, I enjoy bedtime, I dream magical dreams*
- Bedtime is also a good time to use affirmations to reinforce a positive event from that day, to prepare the positive groundwork for the next day or to work on an issue your child may be having i.e. *I am confident, I make friends easily; I am going to do my best today.* You and your child can repeat these affirmations together before they go to sleep
- Using progressive muscle relaxation works really well for children who have trouble winding down. Children can stretch then relax each body part from their toes to their head before settling down for the night

Salt Lamps/House Plants

There are tasteless odourless molecules in the air called ions. They are breathed into our respiratory system. Our technologically dominated homes and workspaces are surrounded with devices that emit large amounts of positive ions into the air when they are in use. Too many positive ions can make us feel tired, depressed and irritable.

Negative ions however make us feel energised and invigorated and some research indicates that they boost the immune system, relieve hay fever and asthma symptoms as well as increase our concentration levels. High concentrations of negative ions are found in forests, bushland, mountains and around beaches and waterfalls.

Salt lamps produce negative ions and improve the air quality. They have wonderful calming and health related properties such as reducing the electromagnetic pollution created by electric equipment and purify the air of dust allergens and even bacteria.

My children have salt lamps in their rooms, which we switch on 15 mins before bedtime. These act as beautiful night lights. I do not profess to be an expert on salt lamps however my family love them and I have a large one in my office and by the children's computer. They certainly create a tranquil atmosphere and look absolutely stunning.

House plants are also a great addition to a home. Plants also produce negative ions. They clean and condition the air adding oxygen and humidity which makes it easier to breath. Some research has shown that air inside the home is more polluted than the air outside. Common house plants can improve air quality by removing toxins, dust particles and other pollutants. These pollutants can contribute to headaches, allergies, asthma, fatigue and many other irritating symptoms. Some of the most popular ones include Boston Ferns, Peace Lilies and Philodendrons.

Your Oasis

How you feel around your home also has a lot to do with your garden and surrounds as well as inside. More plants equals more negative ions which make us feel better. Even if you live in a flat you can pot plants or have an indoor garden. Greenery is magical. Look around your home and find some special places for relaxing. You can make some big throw cushions to chill out on or even put up a hammock. Look in magazines and books for ideas to inspire you. We have a great daybed made out of two recycled packing crates we painted. We covered an old mattress with outdoor fabric and threw a couple of cushions on it. It looks fantastic and is so nice to relax on during summer. Water also has a real calming effect. Ponds or fountains with running water are very relaxing. Again – if you have a small space you can make a water garden in a sealed pot.

Crystals

Crystals are used everyday in modern technology for things such as computers and watches. Crystals are said to have amazing healing properties and many benefits for the body and mind. There are hundreds of books and websites devoted to crystals and they are easily accessible. While they are not for everyone, I have always loved and collected crystals and have several books by Judy Hall on the subject.

Crystals can be used to counteract environmental pollution, in meditation practice, in the bath, in drink bottles, for space cleaning, room cleansing, attracting prosperity, Feng Shui and the list goes on. They can be worn, placed under pillows or even used to make gem essences. Most children love the colours and patterns of crystals and gemstones and the mystique surrounding them. Crystals give my children a magical element to going to sleep at night. They each have a rose quartz crystal by their bed. A lovely lady in a crystal shop told them that if they slept with this under their pillow or by their bed they would have a good night's sleep and peaceful dreams. I also have lepidolite and amethyst by our two computers at home. It is fun to do your own research and explore the world of crystals and how you can use them in your home.

Reading Corner

Setting up a reading corner at home is also a great way to nurture quiet and calm while reinforcing an important skill. Have some big comfy cushions near the book shelf for your children to relax into and read their favourite stories.

Aromatherapy

This is a wonderful therapy to use with children to help create a calm home. Children are born with a great sense of smell. Within days of being born, a baby will recognise his or her own mother by smell alone and their sense of smell increases (just like the sense of taste) as they get older. Different blends of essential oils can be used for all different health issues such as managing stress, relaxation, sleeping better and helping to improve concentration.

Aromatherapy is one of the most magical ways to connect physically, mentally and emotionally. Children respond incredibly well to essential oils either in their bath or vaporiser, in a spritzer, or the most effective way - in a massage. A cup of sea-salt in the bath is also great. Children love it when you take the time to nurture them. Often young children will reject smells, saying they are too strong, so with Aromatherapy it is important to remember that less is best. Only small amounts of essential oils are required in any one application.

I often burn some essential oil, especially lavender or rose geranium at night time in the house and find this very calming. Another favourite is orange oil or lemongrass during the day which I find is very uplifting. We also enjoy using spritzers or room sprays made with essential oil. The fragrance through the house is amazing and some of them are already blended for certain purposes. I love the oils and sprays made by the conscious candle company - www.conscious candle.com.au.

Whilst it is a natural therapy it is important to refer to the experts for recipes and dilutions to ensure you use the right blends. I always use essential oils, be wary of the imitation and synthetic fragrant oils.

One of my favourite books, *Like Chocolate For Women*, has a great pregnancy and children section in it and is full of wonderful information on using aromatherapy for children (full details are in the resource list on Page 280.) You can visit their yummy website www.creativewellbeing.com.

I also use play dough made with added pure essential oils. It influences the senses of touch, smell, and vision and is great for a child's dexterity. It is a fantastic aid to use with children who have Aspergers and Autism.

A selection of the sprays and oils are available at our website **www.indigokidz.com.au**.

Positive Affirmations

At times my kids think I am nuts but I love putting up little affirmations around the house. We have one that says: "Thoughts create things-so think positive thoughts and create positive things". If you have a pin up board or blackboard you can change them weekly. My children each have a set of positive affirmation cards by their bed and all have an artwork in their rooms with empowering words and affirmations. They often choose a card and read it before bedtime which sends them to sleep with a positive thought. It is also important to reinforce positive talk with your children and pick them up when they are being negative and help them rephrase it in a positive light.

Try writing your own affirmations and repeat them throughout the day. Experience the effect it can have first hand. Also be aware of your own language and self talk. Catch yourself when you are saying something in a negative light and rephrase it. This will teach your children to do the same.

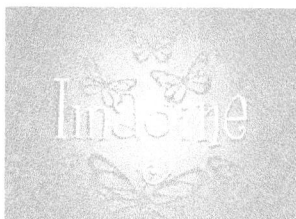

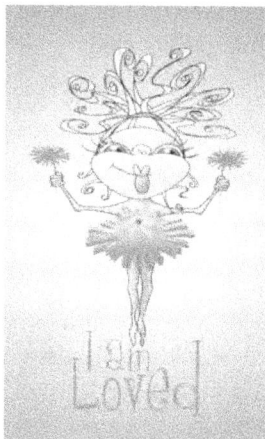

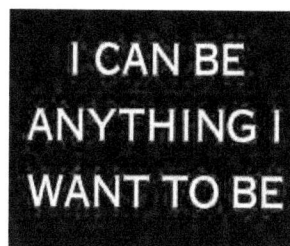

Family Meal and Traditions

No matter what is going on outside the home, families can find a healthy balance by getting back to basics and spending some quality time together. Simple things such as having dinner together with no television on, family game nights, going for bike rides, weekly library visits and family picnics are all part of nurturing a child and creating family time. When I was a child no matter how busy the week was we always had the Sunday night ritual of a roast together. For some families it is a cooked breakfast once a week or dinner together every night at 6pm.

Research suggests that having a regular family meal time promotes communication and relaxation. Children who participate in regular family meals are less likely to be stressed, relate better to people, less likely to participate in risk taking behaviour and are more motivated at school. Saying Grace can be an important part of a family meal ritual. Saying Grace is a wonderful way to express gratitude and does not have to be based on any religion. It can be just a quick thank-you for your family's health and for the meal you are about to eat. Teaching children to be grateful and to express appreciation is an important and often overlooked life skill.

Rituals and traditions give children a sense of stability and belonging. Think back to some of the things you did as children and see if these traditions have been carried on and perhaps start some new ones.

Family Code

Parents have all sorts of ways of keeping peace and order in a home whether it is to help organise homework, chores, pocket money, feeding animals, after school activities or sport.

Creating a family code can be a fun activity that you can all discuss and do together. I also like the sound of code rather than rules. We have a recycling/environment code we have done as a family and also a general one. For the recycling/environment code we looked at ways our family can help the environment and came up with a list including short showers, using the dryer as a last resort, setting up and using our recycling bins, turning all light switches off etc. The kids are all aware and generally do a great job.

Our household code is a little more general and part of it is listed below. I must reiterate that this is for our family only. Your family may have a different view of household behaviour. If your children are aware of the expected behaviour in the house then boundaries are clear:

A Snippet of our Household Code

- Do not harm any living creature
- Kindness always comes back to visit so practice it often
- Honesty is important to all of us as a family
- Always use positive talk and encourage each other
- Manners are magnificent
- Clean up after yourself and always be willing to help as a family member
- Treat our family, home, pets and garden with love and respect
- Respect each other's ideas, opinions, and space
- Quiet time is a good thing that we all need
- Be grateful for our family and for everything we have
- Having things does not make us Happy-Being happy comes from the inside

If children know their boundaries and are part of the decision making process we can all enjoy a happier home environment. The code also ensures that everyone understands the reasons why certain decisions have been made.

Food, Chemicals and Additives

I encourage all parents to read up on all the latest information about chemicals and additives and how they affect their children. Make sure you are aware of what is going into and onto the food you are buying, particularly sugar!

Food additives have been linked to ADHD, cancer, obesity, hindered brain development, rashes, asthma, irritable bowel syndrome, behaviour change and many other ailments. These additives are used to make products taster better, to make the colour appear more vibrant and to thicken watery products. These vibrant colours are used to attract children. I regularly read up on information and share it with my children so that they are also aware.

While we are not focusing on healthy eating I must emphasis that if you want calm centred kids they need to eat a healthy balanced diet full of fresh fruit and vegetables as well as drink plenty of water. I really enjoy the recipes and information in the book "Changing Habits-Changing Lives" by Cyndi O'Meara. It gives easy to read practical advice. Do you own research so you can make informed choices.

It is also important that we are aware of the chemicals that are used in the home. These include cleaning products, shampoo, conditioners, laundry detergents, cling wraps, storage containers, garden sprays and even the water we drink. There are many natural, eco-friendly alternatives these days to help you create a healthy chemical free home environment. There are also many home-made cleaning product recipes using essential oils, bicarbonate soda and vinegar, that are good for you and the environment. Research the information on water filters, use glass containers where possible and try wrapping lunches in recycled brown paper. There are so many alternatives and we have many healthy choices to make. There are some fantastic resources listed at the end of the book.

Vegetable Gardens and Water Tanks

A family vegetable patch teaches children how to grow and care for vegetables and produces fresh, organic produce for the family. You may wish to invest in a water tank so you can water your vegetables with fresh rain water. Learn more about vegetable patches in the "Activities to Nourish your Heart and Soul" section.

Spiritual House Cleaning

Spiritual housecleaning is believed to be a way to get to remove or cleanse negativity or stale energy from your home. Everything that happens within the walls of your house i.e. thoughts, actions, arguments, upsets, illness, guests who have negative energy, previous tenants or owners can upset the balance or your home and leave a negative imprint. People report that following a spiritual houseclean the home feels lighter, safer and much clearer. Listed below are a few of the most popular ways to cleanse your home and make it feel calm and full of positive energy.

Smudging

When we first shifted into our home it had an awful feel or vibe about it. The house felt stale so we smudged it! Smudging is simply the burning of certain herbs to create a fragrant and cleansing smoke which removes negative energy in a house. It is a purification ritual that can be performed in homes, offices, to people or objects. Another common name is sacred smoke bowl blessing. Smudge sticks are often used in Celtic and Native American rituals as part of the traditions and common practice in many traditions. Smudging can also be done after there has been an argument in the house or party where you can have people's energies linger on. Smoke attaches itself to the negative energy and takes it away to be replaced with positive energy. Smudge sticks and instructions for their use are found at most new age shops or on the internet. Make sure you research the properties of any dried herb before using as some herbs can be toxic when burned.

Incense and Candles

You can also use incense sticks for smudging but beware this can set off asthma in some children. Lighting a fragrant candle and allowing the flame to burn away the unwanted energy is also another method for cleansing.

Fresh Air

Opening doors and windows in the house and allowing fresh air to waft through the house is the best way to cleanse a home. Fresh air automatically removes any negativity and stale smells making the house feel clear and light.

Bowl of Water

Many people use a bowl of water kept by the door to help absorb peoples' negative energy and emotions before they enter a house. In some cultures you see the bowls placed at the entrance to a building or home with flowers or candles floating in them. It looks and creates a sense of calm as you come into the house.

Music, Chimes, Bowls and Bells

You can also cleanse your home using the vibration of sound. Sound can cause the atoms in living space to become balanced and harmonious. Sound is used in healing and relaxation and is said to improve physical, mental emotional and spiritual states. Many sounding objects are used in ancient religious practice and rituals such as gongs, temple bells, drums, Tibetan bells, singing bowls, crystal bowls and Tibetan brass bowls. Using sound devices, music or chanting are said to help cleanse a house and remove stale or unwanted energy. It is believed that the sounds emitted resonate throughout the room and drive out any negative energy. You simply walk through each room of your house chiming the bells or striking the bowl using its mallet, banging the drum or chanting. Playing a CD of chanting or playing a sounding device is just as effective for those who are not comfortable with chanting. Yoga and meditation teachers will use sound devices to start and end their practice.

Visualisation

Visualisation is another way of clearing your home. Find a comfortable position, relax and close your eyes. Visualise your home filled with white light that is spreading through each room and washing away any negative or stale energy. Imagine all the dark, heavy energy dissolving in the white light. It is sometimes easy to visualise the white light coming in the front door, moving through each room of the house and going out the back door. You can do this as often as you need to.

Spritzer or Spray

Using a special spritzer or spray in a room can also cleanse your home. As mentioned previously I use the room sprays from the Conscious Candle Company at home and find these not only make the room smell beautiful they lift the feeling in the room. Many of the sprays on the market use different essential oils, herbs and gem essences in them and are made specifically towards removing negativity from a space. You use the spray the same way you would a smudge stick by moving from room to room.

Crystals

Crystals are used in a myriad of ways and one of them is clearing energy. You can place crystals in a bowl anywhere in a room, by the front door or in the corners of rooms. Crystals placed in a bowl not only look beautiful but work to clear negative energy from a room or space. Some of the best crystals for this are Smokey Quartz, Black Obsidian, Snowflake Obsidian, Onyx Apache Tears, Mahogany Obsidian, Citrine and Amethyst. It is important to regularly cleanse your crystals. There are many methods, but the most common include leaving them in the light of a full moon, infusing them with sunlight, burying them in the ground, bathing them in water and sea salt or running them under cool tap water. A great crystal book is the *Crystal Bible* by Judy Hall.

Feng Shui

Another way to bring positive energy and balance into your home is the ancient science of Feng Shui. Feng Shui means "wind" and "water". It is the ancient science of harnessing the naturally occurring life force energies within environment also known as "Chi" to bring good fortune and good health to your home. Feng Shui looks at bringing positive energy flow to your home environment, respecting the integrity of earth and nature, by looking at obstructions, blocks or obstacles within the home. Feng Shui has many rules for successful practice and involves looking at things such as the architecture, interior design, plants, mirrors, windows and grouping of objects within a home environment. There are many consultants now that work in this area. For more information, author Lillian Too is an expert in the field. Her book "Total Feng Shui: Bring Health, Wealth and Happiness into Your Life", is a great resource.

Creating a Calm Study Space

Although younger children generally do not have homework they certainly benefit from having a calm study space when doing projects. Good habits will carry through to the teenage years where creating a calm study space is even more important.

Here are a few tips:

- A workspace to be used just for study with a comfortable chair
- The study space should be clear, organised and clutter free
- Pencils, pens and other equipment stored in an easy to reach container
- Use labels, magazine holders and files so everything is easily found and accessible
- Make sure the room has good ventilation and plenty of light
- Have a salt lamp nearby and turn it on while they are working
- Have a living plant near the desk or study area
- Play some calming background music in the room if your child is easily distracted by general household noise
- Encourage your child to take a few deep breaths before commencing their study or project

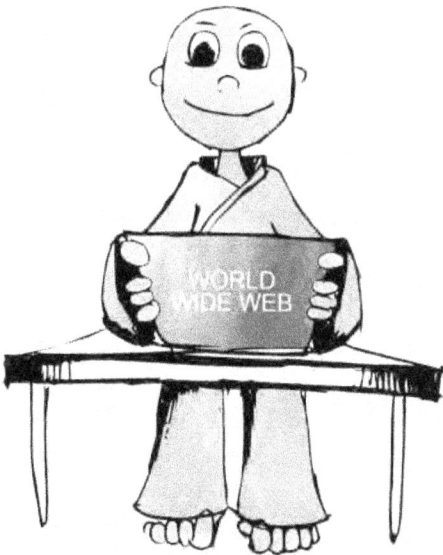

Connected to the
world wide web

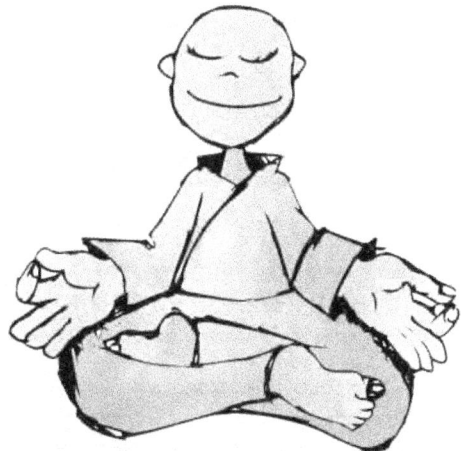

Connected to the
universal web

Ideas to Create a Calm Home

- Be calm yourself. Children pick up on your stress. Remember being calm is contagious
- Regularly cleanse your house and practice spiritual housecleaning
- Have an organised, clutter-free home
- Have a relaxing bedtime routine
- Use salt lamps around computers and in bedrooms
- Get outdoors, create a vegetable patch and get some herbs growing
- Fill your home with positive affirmations, quotes and uplifting messages
- Have some living plants in the house-great air purifiers
- Create your own oasis with garden and potted plants
- Use oils and sprays in your home
- Set up some family rituals and traditions
- Work on a household code
- Express gratitude often
- Make a relaxation space or area in your house
- Give your children time to just "be" and to relax!
- Get outside and make some great experiences for you and your family-check out all the activities in the "Nurturing Your Heart and Soul" Chapter
- Stop and take some deep breaths every hour. Take care of you! Nurture yourself, lots of sleep, exercise regularly
- Work out some ground rules for the use of technology and social networking as a family

Calm Home = Calm Parents, Calm Parents = Calm Kids

Teaching Meditation and Relaxation at Home

How you teach meditation in your home relies on what you as a parent feel comfortable with and your family dynamics, this is a guide only. Do what you feel is right and what works in your home. I have outlined some information for parents based on the questions I am most frequently asked. I have also added in some of my family's personal practices.

Please don't imagine that my house is a constantly serene place where everyone is completely centred and focused all the time. My kids argue and fight and are at times completely unreasonable. I often find myself trying to scream louder than them. When this happens, we try to take a few deep breaths together. I love the fact that my children are free spirited. They love trying new things and are generally aware of their environment and of what goes on around them. They know how to calm themselves, are confident, compassionate and mindful in their daily lives.

Some Benefits of Teaching Meditation and Relaxation at Home

- Provides a great bonding opportunity
- Increases family communication
- Bedtime becomes fun and not stressful
- Gives parents a chance to participate in the experience and to relax
- Provides a calm atmosphere in the house
- Teaches children and parents how to have quiet time
- Provides a tool to handle emotions and feelings in a positive way
- It can provide a wonderful insight into your children
- Provides an opportunity to share feelings and emotions
- Teaches the whole family how to just "be" rather than having to "do"

Special Place

You can set up a special place for meditation or relaxation activities in any home. Children may like to create their own special space or you may use a specific room away from the hustle and bustle in the household. If you are lucky enough to have a dedicated room at home you may like to paint it a peaceful colour such as soft green or blue. You may wish to use cushions or blankets for comfort. You may like to create a meditation altar using flowers, crystals, candles, a favourite picture, incense or other objects to promote a sense of peace and tranquillity. Your children will then associate this quiet place with meditation.

You can sit facing your child (or in a circle if you have more than one child) and complete the meditation lying on the floor or when they are in their bed so they can drift off into a peaceful sleep. Make sure that you have limited interruptions from such things as mobile phones. You may find that even the family pet may try and get in on the act. Our dog likes nothing better than to be with us at meditation time and has learned to lie quietly on the floor next to us. Of course not all pets will do this and may need to be put outside or in another room.

How Often

Meditating at a similar time each day helps with the preparation. If they are really tired or have trouble settling at night, then I do the meditation in bed so they can relax and fall asleep afterwards.

Ideally it would be great if children could meditate every day, but I realise that this is not always possible. I am often asked how I meditate at home when I have three children of differing ages and differing commitments. I use a combination of CD's and visualisations from a book. My younger children generally go to bed at night listening to relaxing music or a meditation CD. Their favourite relaxation CD is *Dream of the Dolphins* by *Serenity.* The combination of music and the sounds of nature work wonders. One night a week we meditate together before bedtime. We sit in a circle and choose a meditation from a book or I tap into a bit of creativity and explore my own imagination (often at the end of the day it is sadly lacking). My children love to do a warm up activity to start and it helps to balance their energy. Sometimes we discuss a problem or issue that one of them brings up and this is a cue for the type of meditation we do or we pick a relaxation exercise or calming technique. My teenage son now chooses to do his own thing but I am confident that he has a full tool kit he can tap into as the need arises.

Meditation and some of the techniques involved can be used in the home environment anytime, not just at night time. If a child is upset, overstimulated, and angry or if you simply feel they will benefit from it, use some of the calming techniques or breathing exercises followed by a calming visualisation. Calming techniques are very useful for children who are faced with exams. Meditation as a family is more challenging because it takes a little more planning and perseverance but the benefits are well worth the initial effort.

Sharing Time

When a family meditates together it is important for the discussions to be open and honest. It may be good a time to discuss worries, issues or concerns that have arisen within the family. Meditation together as a family affair can offer great insight in to the family dynamics. It provides uninterrupted time together where you all have each other's undivided attention. Not all members of the family may wish to be involved. I suggest making them aware it is important to respect the quiet time and to read, draw or listen to some music quietly until the rest of the family has finished. As children get older they may wish to meditate on their own or find their own methods of relaxing and meditation. After the meditation the family can share their thoughts and feelings. This can help to keep lines of communication open.

Outside - Mindful Meditation

I always encourage my children and any children I am teaching to just be still for a few moments if they are outside in nature. If they are in a park or at the beach watching a sunset, encourage your children to take in some deep breaths and listen to the sounds of nature all around them. Encourage them to watch the colours of the sunset, look at nature's many colours and enjoy the surroundings. Encourage them to close their eyes, listen, feel, breathe, smell and take it all in. This is a mini meditation. Taking your family hiking or bushwalking or walking along the beach, especially at sunset, is a form of mindful meditation. Stop every so often and take in the beauty that surrounds you. Fresh air and nature are great for recharging the system and help us escape the noise and pace of daily life. It is such a simple thing that we often don't remember to stop and do.

Technology

Technology is a huge part of our modern world and it is only going to keep advancing. It has made some groundbreaking and positive differences to our world while also creating its own set of unique problems. I am often asked if I ban my children from electronics and games and the simplest explanation I give is to remind people that technology is going to play an even greater role in the future. Our kids are growing up in this age of development so I try and integrate it into our lives and teach my children how to cope with its influence. I think it is important not to forget the basics and to teach them how to find their own sense of calm within, rather than react to the external influences of technology. It is important that they get outside, have experiences and spend time each day in some form of unstructured outdoor play or activity. My husband and I limit their time on electronic devices and try to discuss the reasons why. All our electronics go into a special cupboard at night out of the children's rooms. As a family we have set our ground rules but as parents we have made the time to actively engage our children in the world around them.

I suggest that as parents we monitor the use of social media and keep communication open. Each family will have its own unique circumstances and I believe that discussing it together and devising a plan for your family is the best way. As adults we need to be aware of the effects of passive entertainment and teach our children how to interact in the real world with real people and real friends.

There are many great images that encapsulate this mindset. I recently saw a picture of an empty swing set titled "The Original Play Station-Get Real Get Outside". These images are definitely food for thought.

Spiritual

Meditation need not be contrary to anyone's religious or spiritual beliefs. You may incorporate your beliefs into the visualisations, discussions and awareness activities. When meditating at home you can use part of your meditation routine to offer a special message for someone, for example a sick relative. You can use this time to say thank you for everything the family has, or to discuss a teaching, prayer or topic based on your family's beliefs.

Meditation Manners

These are very important at home as children often are "themselves" in all their wonderful glory and may not act like they do in a school situation. It is important to discuss your motives and reasons why you would like to introduce meditation or relaxation practices into your home and discuss all the benefits with your child. You may wish to discuss *Meditation Manners* outlined in the chapter *Meditation for the First Time*.

Meditation as an Individual

You may find older children who become familiar with the practice of meditation and its benefits, may like to do it on their own. If you do not have a designated space in the house you may like to help them prepare one in their room. Meditation is a great way to refresh and refocus when studying. My eldest son (who loves sports) uses a form of meditation prior to any big sporting events to help him stay calm. He visualises himself performing the sport or skill successfully. It really helps him as it acts like a mental rehearsal. I have spoken to other children in upper primary school who use visualisation when they are feeling confused or out of sorts. One child meditated when they felt bored and found that afterwards they always came up with a new and fresh idea.

As children become more familiar with meditation you may find that they want to lead the meditation themselves or come up with their own visualisation. They may not be able to offer a full visualisation but it is important to encourage your child and participate with them. My daughter likes to lead us and sometimes it is very hard to wipe the smile off my face. She uses a very heavenly voice and although sometimes the journey is a little disjointed she really has a good handle on the concept and it becomes a special time for us all.

Suggested Practice for Meditation at Home

This suggested outline for meditation practice takes about 10 to 15 minutes and is a guide only. It is important to do what feels right for you and your family. Often people who follow a routine find it easier to reach a meditative state as they are already making the mind-body connection during the preparation. You can make up your own meditations according to interests and needs. You can even record them onto a CD for your children to listen to at night. You then have another alternative and your children go to bed listening to a very friendly and familiar voice. This is a great choice for when you are out and have a babysitter who can switch it on for your kids.

Suggested Outline for Practicing Meditation at Home

- Prepare for your meditation i.e. quiet room, comfortable clothing, eliminate potential distractions
- Find your comfortable position
- Practice one of the activities listed in the book as a fun warm-up
- Start to focus on the breath. Take 5-10 deep breaths to prepare
- Repeat the affirmation 3- 5 times (if using an affirmation to focus)
- Beginning sequence
- Begin the meditation *(visualisation)*
- Leave children in the meditation at the open-ended section for a few minutes (if in bed you may wish to leave them to drift off to sleep at this point and repeat the affirmation here)
- End the meditation with the closing sequence
- Repeat the affirmation (if using an affirmation)
- Discussion or artwork/journal

Parent Experiences

Here are some personal stories from parents who have used meditation and relaxation with their children.

Experience 1

Fiona is a mother of two children, a seven year old girl who has anxiety issues and a five year old boy who is so relaxed that she describes him as a big lump of floppy jelly. Fiona has been using meditation herself for years and thought it might help her daughter with her anxiety. Fiona uses meditation in two ways, which she describes below:

Bedtime: I will often read them a story and then we do a meditation from Indigo Dreaming. I've told my son if he doesn't want to do it he just has to lie still and quiet and let us do it. It is taking some time to get them to concentrate on their breathing. I don't answer their questions or respond to them during the meditation at all. I wait until the end. I go through the meditation and although my son says he doesn't want to do it I hear him whisper answers to all the questions asked. Eg Magic Mirror - Can you see the beautiful purple, velvet drapes with the big gold sashes? No. You walk over to the mirror. The mirror is as tall as you and encrusted with beautiful crystals of all colours. What colours can you see? Blue and Red. I don't hear my daughter answer but I have asked her and she has said that she can imagine what I am saying. Usually at the end of a night time meditation she is very relaxed and sleepy.

Before School: I try to do a quick meditation before school. I choose one with an affirmation appropriate to whatever situation they are facing at school at the time. I've found since using the meditation that in times of stress my daughter will start to use the breathing techniques to calm her self down. She loves the visualisations and messages provided by the meditations. She particularly likes the idea of the Magic Worry Hat. I'm hoping that in time she will use this hat at school when she is worried about things. I've asked my daughter what she likes about the meditations: "They're fantastic, I love them. I like the stories."

Experience 2

Lisa is a 42 year old mother of two children aged 13 and 10. Lisa uses meditation in place of reading a story at night time to settle her engergetic 10 year old son. Lisa discusses:

My 10 year old son quite often gets his second wind right at bed time and says to me "I'm not tired Mum" and "I have lots of energy Mum" as he wriggles around the bed. I pull out the book of meditations and am not even half through the beginning routine when I see him starting to calm and settle down. He knows the procedure, he closes his eyes, breathes in and out and it is like the ants in his pants have left.

The affirmations he learns and imagines in the stories offer a topic for discussion and are reinforced in everyday activities. My son likes me to read several of the visualisations each night. I am lucky to make it through two visualisations before he is asleep peacefully. Using meditation settles him in such a short period of time. For a little boy who, like most children these days, is over stimulated all day, it is lovely to spend such quiet, peaceful and precious time with him doing a valuable and creative activity.

❀ Experience 3

Jessica is a mother of two young children aged four and seven. Her seven year old son Jake has been the source of much soul searching in their family unit. This is Jessica's story:

My son Jake has not had an easy time at school. He struggles to listen and concentrate in class. He never seems to complete any tasks and is at times quite anti establishment, so to speak. I have been to therapists, doctors and specialists. He has trouble settling at night and our house has become quite stressful. He was diagnosed with ADHD and it was recommended that my son begin taking medication. I understand that for some families this is their journey and the medication may be needed but I decided against it and looked for alternatives.

First I looked at diet and additives to make sure I was giving Jake the best nutrition I could. A friend suggested that I started teaching Jake meditation. I began by letting him listen to a CD and then through to reading meditations from a book. He responded better doing the meditation with me and I enjoyed it too as it seemed to make me more relaxed. I found the best time to do meditation was at bed time with a book. At first Jake would wriggle around and talk and say he was bored and that it was stupid. I persevered and after a few weeks found that he wriggled less and less and was actually lying still with his eyes closed listening to me. He now asks to do a meditation at bed time. I noticed he would say comments like, "I love going to the quiet beach, and I have friends there". This made me realise that he was actually visualising.

I noticed a few small changes in Jake over the weeks, bedtime was much easier and he seemed to be much calmer and more relaxed. One of his teachers commented that he had really improved in class and that he was less distracted. This was further validation of what I was already starting to see at home. I continue to work with Jake, teaching him how to relax, understand his feelings and not to lash out. Meditation has made a huge difference and I am so grateful that I stayed with it and did not turn to medication to help with his behaviour. Putting in the effort, having loads of patience and spending that quiet time together was worth it. I also benefit from the quiet time together and am learning to use meditation myself. It has made a huge difference to our family and to the quality time I now spend with my daughter.

❀ Experience 4

Leanne is a working mother of energetic twin boys. Leanne uses a combination of meditations from a book and guided meditation CD's. This is her story;

As a working mother of two, at the end of the day I am always tired and a little irritable! I find it difficult to remain relaxed and calm as bedtime approaches. I have twin boys who are always excitable and over active right around bed time. I would get a little crankier than I wanted to and would just want to put them to bed. I always read to the boys at bedtime but decided to try something a little different - meditation. A friend had written a wonderful meditation book so I decided to give it a try.

Initially the boys thought it was very funny lying there with their eyes closed and imagining things. They started to giggle and couldn't stop. I had to try a new approach so I would take one at a time off to a quiet comfortable room and read to them individually. As time went by and the boys became used to the routine I could read to them both at the same time without the fear of a giggling marathon. The boys then began requesting certain meditations that were their favourites and I began choosing ones that were relevant to what was happening in their lives. If they had certain behavioural issues that needed dealing with, I would choose a meditation relevant to that issue.

We also have a CD with the meditations on that I use on long car trips. When the boys start getting a little bored or restless on goes the CD. They are instantly quiet and attentively listening to the storyteller. One of my boys in particular will often drift off to sleep. The book is also handy on holidays particularly if there are other children around making bedtime even more of a chore. The book comes out and the boys slowly relax at the end of a very exciting day.

We started meditation when the boys were four and they are now nearly seven. They still enjoy drifting of into the land of imagination. We don't read meditations every night but maybe once or twice a week alternating with storybooks to keep things interesting.

In the future I would like to get my husband involved and start doing some family meditation as, like all families, our lives and busy and we need to slow down even it is for just a few minutes a day.

⬡ Experience 5

Donna is a mother of two children, Matt aged five and Hayley who is eight. Donna has used the visualisations with her children and shares her story below:

I initially looked for children's meditation for Hayley. She is quite a busy person both physically and emotionally. I have used meditation myself on and off for about 20 years so I was well aware of the benefits of it. I'm quite partial to visualisations myself so to find a book which was written for children was really like finding a pot of gold. Matt was initially reluctant to do it but he is now very keen. Usually we do our meditation at night. Over time the kids have learnt to lie still and listen and wait till the end if they have any questions. We've been using the meditations for about a year now so they've learned to answer the questions asked in their head now rather than out loud. I get the two of them to lie down and I dim the lights. Sometimes I will put on relaxation music in the background but not always.

We do the meditation and I always give them time at the end to lie still and think about the message. I find that after doing the meditation they are always nice and calm and relaxed. I do believe that it helps the kids to have an active imagination, which I believe to be vitally important. I also believe that it helps their self-belief and self confidence, something that was lacking.

Meditation is something that I will continue to do with them and I hope they will use it themselves throughout their lives.

Teaching Meditation and Relaxation in Schools

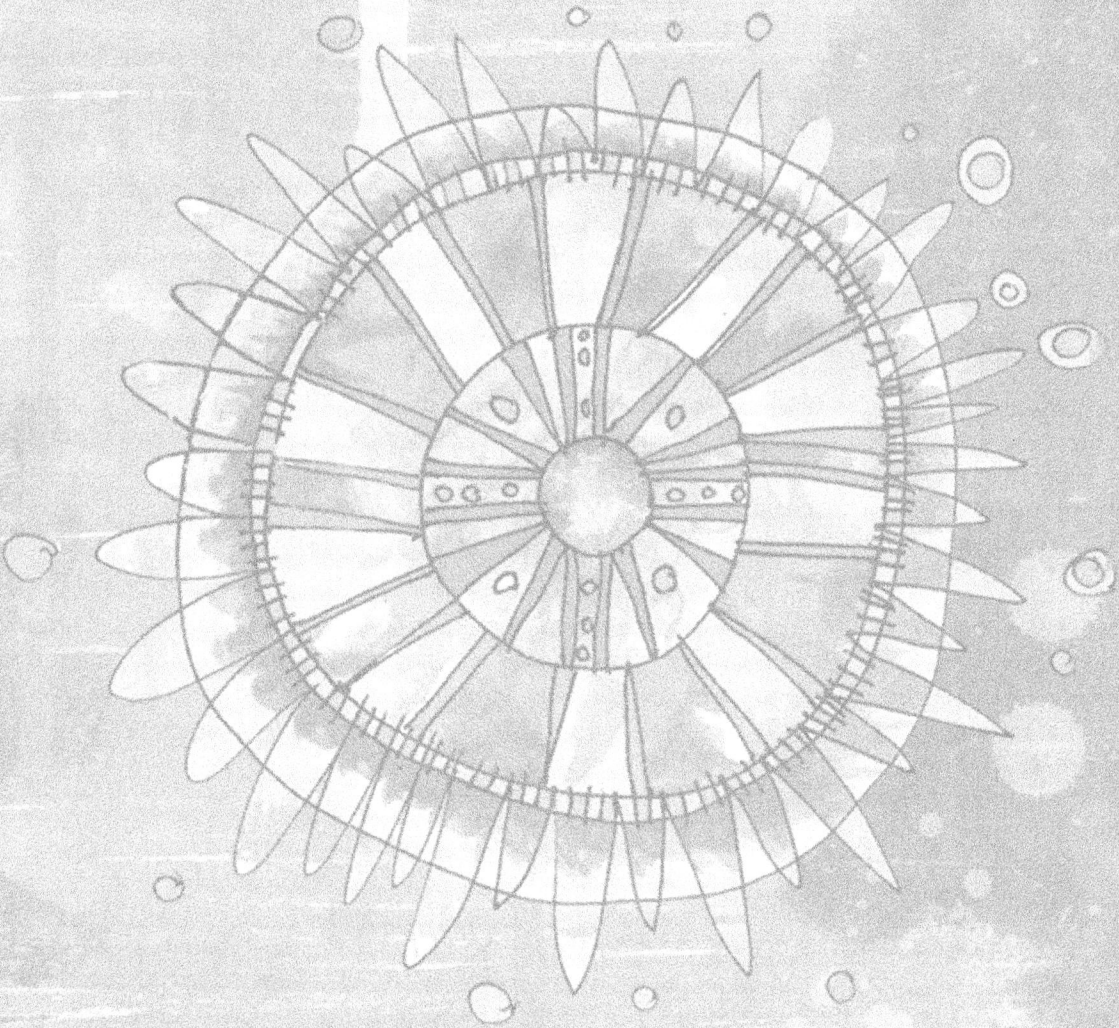

Creating a Calm Classroom

Teachers are simply amazing! Not many other jobs have to contend with up to 30 or more people in their office or workspace all day long, five days a week. Primary teachers normally have a designated classroom and can create their own space. Secondary teachers often move from room to room but can use some of the tips below. Some teachers have remote students so the computer becomes their classroom! Here are a few tips to help you to be a calm teacher and to create a calm classroom.

Walk the Walk

I have repeated some of this paragraph from creating a calm home because it applies to all adults who are trying to help children to be calm and relaxed. We must remember that our stress can influence children and that we are the role models from whom they watch and learn.

Be mindful of your voice tone, your breathing and posture while teaching. Take time to meditate yourself or try some of the calming strategies in this book. Taking three minutes a day to do deep breathing is a great start. A great calming technique for teachers is to stop and remember to take five deep breaths every hour. Sounds simple and yet such a simple activity can bring enormous rewards to our lives.

Class Rules and your Teaching Style

All classrooms have rules and all teachers have individual teaching styles. Teachers are great at letting their classes know the rules and formulating them together is a good process. If boundaries are clearly set, then children know what is expected of them. Children will soon learn what type of teacher you are and your style of teaching, so add calm from the beginning!

Declutter and Organise

I am a firm believer in clutter-free homes and classrooms. Many experts point to the benefits of de-cluttering and point out that an organised home or office is more peaceful. When moving from room to room it is not always easy to remain clutter-free, however you can keep your office desk or work area organised. Give everything a home in a labelled box or tray. Not only are they easier to find but you will be able to easily transport materials from class to class or to desks for lessons. Get students to help you clean out and get organised. It is always a good activity to do in the last days of school as you get ready for next year and there is a bit more down time.

Salt Lamps/Plants

Please refer to the information in *Teaching Meditation and Relaxation at Home* - Creating a Calm Home, on Page 74. Our technologically dominated homes and workspaces are filled with devices that emit large amounts of positive ions into the air when they are in use. Salt Crystal lamps have wonderful calming and health-related properties such as reducing the electromagnetic pollution created by electric equipment and purifying the air of dust allergens and even bacteria. If you have your own classroom you can easily have a salt lamp on your desk or at the back of the classroom. You might also include Indoor plants or even a small bunch of fresh flowers, which can liven up a classroom. Bring the outside in and let the kids enjoy it.

Fish Tanks

Fish tanks are very therapeutic. There is something very calming about watching fish swimming about. It also teaches the children how to take care of a pet. Many doctors' surgeries and waiting rooms have them for this purpose.

Quiet Corner

Setting up a reading corner in a classroom is also a great way to nurture quiet and calm while reinforcing an important skill. Have some big comfy cushions near the book shelf for the children who finish their work early to relax into and read their favourite stories.

Calm Corner/Calm Down Kit

When teaching you can often get a child who is very stressed or anxious and needs to be calmed down whilst you are still trying to work with the remaining class members. If you have a *Calm Down Kit* in your quiet corner you can use this as a tool for the child to cope with anxiety or anger. You will need a box and then you can work with your students on some ideas of what to put in the box. Things such as noise cancelling head phones, relaxing books, stress ball, play dough, laminated pictures of peaceful scenes, sea shells, feathers, finger mazes and sensory jars. You can have some relaxing music and headphones ready to go. Calm boxes work very well especially if students are involved in the process of putting them together. (Visit **www.indigokidz. com.au** for more information on making Calm Down Kits.)

Aromatherapy

This is a wonderful therapy to help create a calm home or classroom. Please refer to *Teaching Meditation and Relaxation at Home* - Creating a Calm Home, on Page 74 for more information, but recognise that children generally respond well to essential oils in a vaporiser or in a spritzer. However not all schools would be happy with teachers who had oil burners in their classroom so check with your principal first. Electric oil burners are best so there are no candles burning. You also need to be aware of those with asthma and allergies! It seems a big checklist. I like to use lavender, orange and lemon in a class. Lavender is calming and orange and lemon are meant to be uplifting and good for studying. We all know what classrooms can smell like at times and it is not pleasant. Another way to keep your classroom fresh is to use a fragrant spray that has essential oils. I suggest a quick spray first thing in the morning before the kids come in and then again before they come back from lunch.

I also use play dough with essential oils in a class situation. Again, you will find more information on this product in *Teaching Meditation and Relaxation at Home* - Creating a Calm Home, on Page 74. It is good to use with kinaesthetic learners and for children who are struggling to settle into meditation. Holding it in their hand to touch stops them fidgeting and squirming and helps to calm them. It is a fantastic aid for teachers to use with children with ADHD, Asperger's and Autism.

A selection of the sprays and oils are available at our website **www.indigokidz.com.au**.

Positive Affirmations

I love putting up little affirmations around the house, in my office and in a classroom. You can decorate your classroom with lots of positive messages or have children make their own. There are plenty of ideas in the activities section at the end of the book. If you are moving from class to class you can use positive speech to remind children how special they are. Make it a point each class to pick out a child and give them some positive feedback. As a teacher, if I hear a child using negative talk, I try and alert them to the fact and help them to rephrase it. Children that I have taught know this about me and I constantly reinforce that if they keep saying it they will program their mind to believe it-so program your mind with positive talk instead! Positive comments from teachers can make a child's day so dish out as many as you can.

Posters of nature and serene scenes can also add to a calm classroom atmosphere. Sunsets, rainforests, tropical beaches, rainbows and waterfalls can add a bit of magic to any classroom.

Take Care of Yourself

I would like a dollar for every time I've heard "what a great life teachers have and how do they get stressed out with so many holidays." Teachers need to take care of themselves and although this is basic stuff, it is easily forgotten. Take time to nurture yourself in your downtime with a regular massage or body treatment. Try a warm bath, yoga or some daily exercise to help you unwind. As with children, getting a good night's sleep is so important. If you have trouble sleeping try some of the calming strategies in this book.

Work out a set of daily affirmations just for you and repeat them throughout the day. Cut down the tea and coffee and drink plenty of water throughout the day. I always have a water bottle at hand when teaching. Eating healthy meals helps to keep your energy levels up and also aids your immune system. Teachers are faced with a variety of bugs and germs courtesy of the children they teach and it is important to stay stress free and healthy so they don't succumb to them.

Perhaps most importantly, remember to practice what you preach and try some visualisation and meditation practice. Try all the different activities for yourself and use your favourite ones often!

Check out the *Teaching Meditation and Relaxation at Home* Chapter as well. There is some information on using sound and clearing energy that some teachers may wish to read and much of the information is transferable. Also, if you are a practitioner who deals with children there are many points from both sections that will be relevant to your work environment.

Summary - How to Create a Calm Classroom

- Be calm. Children pick up on teacher stress. Remember being calm is contagious
- Use a quiet calm voice
- Be clutter free
- Be organised
- Fill your class with posters of positive affirmations, quotes, uplifting messages or beautiful serene scenes
- Use positive talk in your class and develop some affirmations just for you
- A fish tank in the classroom can be very therapeutic
- Living plants in the classroom-great air purifiers

- Use oils and sprays in your class
- Manage your time effectively - the more productive you are the less stressed you are
- Have regular breaks when teaching, get out in the fresh air when you can
- Eat healthy meals. Bring plenty of fruit to snack on during the day
- Have a water bottle on your desk or to take from class to class
- Try not to drink tea or coffee at work. Try herbal teas
- Stop and take some deep breaths every hour. Take care of you! Nurture yourself, lots of sleep, exercise regularly

Calm teacher = Calm Classroom
Calm Classroom = Optimal Learning Environment

Teaching Meditation and Relaxation in Schools

I am frequently asked to speak at schools and to groups of teachers on meditation and relaxation activities for students. Meditation has gained widespread acceptance in the medical profession as a tool for relaxation and to combat stress. Visualisation is used with great success in the business, sports and health industries, yet these practices are still a relatively new teaching tool in the classroom.

Teachers are under more pressure than ever in the classroom. They have a changing curriculum, administrative demands, parents to deal with, children with behavioural problems and learning disorders. Children are coming to school already exhausted, often without breakfast and suffering from lack of sleep. Pressure to achieve on national tests, children on medication, split level classes, children with developmental issues and the list goes on! There is no doubt in my mind that most teachers are probably suffering the side effects of negative stress on a daily basis.

Teachers have no control over what happens to a child outside the classroom. However if we can help children to recognise the symptoms of stress and provide them with tools to help deal with it, then we are helping to make a more centred child who can take this knowledge and apply it outside the classroom.

Creating an Optimal Learning Environment

Meditation has been long favoured for its health benefits but it can also compliment the process of learning. Children learn more effectively and absorb more information when they are relaxed and focused. Meditation and calming techniques can help to produce this mentally alert state. If a teacher has a relaxed, calm class children will enjoy the learning process. Although in its infancy, researchers are investigating the effects of meditation on children who have behavioural and developmental learning disorders and problems with concentration and focus.

A study of college students in the US showed that students who regularly meditated had a higher grade-point average, increased self esteem, decreased psychological distress, less aggressive behaviour, better work habits, better class attendance records, and decreased lateness attending class. Another study revealed that students who study relaxation techniques have fewer days of absenteeism and suspensions. As interest in the field of meditation and education increases, more research will be produced leading to a wider acceptance of meditation in schools and colleges.

Note: **For more information and research on Meditation and Schools I recommend** *Meditation in Schools - Calmer Classrooms* **by Clive and Jane Erricker, Gina Levete.**

Benefits for Teachers

Meditation can enhance a student's enjoyment of learning while helping teachers improve the classroom environment in which they work. Here are a few important facts:

- Meditation creates an optimal learning environment
- Gives teachers a chance to participate in the experience
- Gives teachers some quiet, calm time
- Children become calmer and more attentive
- Enjoyable for the teacher and the students
- Provides a focus for other classroom activities
- Provides a non-threatening way to explore important issues
- It can help to settle a class
- Students are more self aware
- It can help to rejuvenate and refocus
- It is cost effective and no special equipment is required
- It does not require a large amount or preparation time
- It is easy to slot into a teaching timetable
- It can provide a great stimulus for creative activities

Research has shown there to be less aggression, better behaviour, less truancy, a decrease in bullying and an improvement in school work with classes participating in a regular meditation program.

Why teachers don't teach Meditation or Relaxation Activities

The most common statements I hear from teachers are;

- I am not trained
- I can't fit it into an already impossible schedule,
- Parents will think we are "crazy" teaching it
- The principal won't allow it
- We don't teach religious based programs

Most of these points have been discussed in *About Meditation* and I hope this book has helped clarify the benefits and inspire you to have the confidence and tools to begin teaching meditation. If you take 10 minutes a day and make it part of your daily routine, I am sure you will see a more productive class with higher levels of focus, concentration and the ability to stay on task. It would be great to see meditation as part of the whole school ethos and included daily.

Principal/Parent Permission

I have heard teachers say that they teach meditation under the term *Relaxation Time* so that they do not upset parents or the principal. I personally always use *Meditation* and educate parents, teachers and principals about the term, benefits and the objectives I am trying to achieve with the children.

I suggest discussing these objectives with parents at the start of the year in your first parent meeting. Outline the benefits and the reason you are teaching meditation. I also discuss the process and how I incorporate visualisation, calming strategies and other activities such as body awareness and focusing. If need be, invite your principal or parents in to watch your class practice, so they can see what you are doing with the children. Most principals and parents tend to be very receptive and supportive of anything that aids the process of learning. Be aware that some principals may ask you to obtain parental permission.

Children who Struggle to Concentrate

Children who struggle the most with meditation are the ones who have difficulty settling down and paying attention in general. However these students are also the ones that you often see the biggest improvements in and that need meditation the most. Teachers report to me that after participating in meditation, children's stories and artwork became more colourful, creative and with finer detail. It is as if the door to the imagination has opened wide. Meditation encourages children to focus and concentrate and provides a fun, relaxing way in which to improve in this area.

School Set Up

You may be lucky enough to have a large room you can use in the school or otherwise may simply have to use the space in your classroom. It is a good idea to have a clear, uncluttered space that is well ventilated, but this is not always practical or possible. Teachers are excellent at finding space when needed and with a few desks and chairs moved out of the way it should be quick and easy. Remember any of these activities can also be done at a school desk!

You may do it with your whole class or it may be something that is done with groups. It may be that one teacher who has an interest, moves throughout the school taking various groups. It would be ideal if each teacher could take their own class as they have built a relationship with them.

One teacher reported using meditation with a group of children with learning difficulties. They were taken from class to participate in a small group and it was having a noticeable affect on their concentration and focus in their normal class activities.

Timing

You only need 10 to 15 minutes a day. If you can't do it each day, try to offer it two or three times a week and on the other days do a few minutes deep breathing. The more often children participate in meditation, the greater the benefits for both students and teacher. A good time to offer meditation is usually first thing in the morning or immediately after lunch. If you do your meditation at a similar time each day then you will find children will prepare much more quickly. If your class is restless throughout the day or lacking energy, stop what you are doing and do a mini meditation or some breathing activities to rejuvenate and re focus them. The one minute recharge is great to use after each break in the school day to refocus children and turn their relaxation response back on.

Some of the schools in the United Kingdom, who are seeing some fantastic results from regular meditation, are doing two ten minute sessions each day.

Schools and Religion

Meditation is an important element within all the great spiritual traditions and is vital to strengthening faith and belief. It is my opinion, and that of many leaders in the field of children's meditation, that meditation should be taught to young children without a particular set of beliefs being expressed unless the school operates within a recognised religious framework or the school is based on the philosophy and spiritual values of the schools' founders.

A "new age" approach should be avoided in mainstream schools. These techniques are best saved for groups organised out of school that have the full support of parents or guardians. As a child matures and becomes experienced at meditation he or she will be able to make their own decisions. Older children can try the different types and approaches to meditation and explore some of the rich philosophies in which it is based.

Preparation

It is a good idea to have the area ready before hand. This is not always possible and moving chairs and tables can be noisy, but if it is done as part of the preparation before each session, children will get used to it and it will become part of the routine. It is a good idea to get children into a routine from the moment they begin. If you do meditation each day following lunch then get children in the practice of taking their shoes off outside, they then come in, get a rug or pillow (if you have them), find a space and are ready to go. Several teachers I have spoken to have the relaxing music already playing as a cue for the children. The children now go about their preparation without any prompt from the teachers at all.

A school in the United Kingdom has special mediation room in the school with a meditation/relaxation club timetable supervised and supported by the teaching staff. In addition the school has identified a group of students with various behaviour and/ or learning difficulties who attend meditation regularly. The program has been reported as a great success with parents and teachers all witnessing improvements in behaviour and ability to concentrate and focus in class.

When I was teaching I would take my oil burner and lavender oil to class. It would take a few seconds to set up and I kept it safely away from the children. Now they have electric oil burners which are very safe and easy to use. The students loved it and it helped to make a special classroom atmosphere.

Children Leading the Visualisation

Older children often like to write their own visualisations. Not only is it a creative writing exercise but a fantastic exercise for self-expression, speaking and reading skills. You can try a different one each week and discuss it afterwards. This is a great exercise for the imagination, as the child will need to visualise their scenario and then put it on paper.

Suggested Meditation Practice for a School

This is a suggested outline for doing a meditation or relaxation session in a school setting. It would take 10-15 minutes. Remember this is a guide only. Do what feels right for you and your class. You can make up your own meditations according to the interests and needs of your students or you may wish to have a class theme or topic. Some days you may wish to do a mini meditation, a relaxation activity or a meditation from a CD. Variety makes it interesting as long as the routine is similar and that they are doing some calming breathing as part of the process.

Suggested Outline for a Class Meditation Practice (approx. 15 minutes)

- Prompt to start meditation practice i.e. spoken prompt, ring a triangle or bell. Early childhood classes often have pillows for children to use or you may have a set of class mats or blankets that they get ready
- Ask the child to find a comfortable position, let them experiment until they are comfortable
- Quick reminder of class meditation manners
- Practice one of the activities listed in the book as a fun warm-up.
- Start to focus on the breath, do 5-10 deep breaths to prepare
- Repeat the affirmation 3- 5 times (if doing a meditation with an affirmation)
- Beginning sequence
- Begin the meditation (Visualisation)
- Leave children in the meditation at the open ended section (depending on class and teacher's timetable) for a few minutes
- End the meditation with the closing sequence
- Repeat the affirmation (if using one)
- Discussion and/or follow up activity

Teacher Experiences

Here are some personal stories from classroom teachers who have used meditation with their children.

Experience 1 - Annette

Annette is a teacher with 30 years experience who is currently teaching years 3 and 4 in a metropolitan primary school. Annette has been meditating herself for approximately 15 years and began teaching meditation in a primary school setting approximately 6 years ago.

Annette practices meditation with her class every day immediately following the lunch break. The meditation lasts for approximately 15-20 minutes and then the class participates in silent reading. Annette also uses meditation to focus her class first thing in the morning if she feels her class are "scatty".

The meditation practice consists of deep breathing and relaxation, followed by a visualisation that is guided. Annette uses a combination of CD's and reading the visualisations from a book. Follow-up activities take place as part of the health and wellbeing strand in the curriculum. Her school principal is supportive of meditation and no parental permission was required. She is currently the only teacher in the school teaching meditation but reports that other teachers have been asking how they teach it after seeing how calm and focused her teaching environment is. The school is looking to introduce it across all grades next year after seeing its positive effects.

Annette reports that if she is away from class and they have a relief teacher, the students will tell the relief teacher that they do meditation everyday and show the teacher the books and CD to use. She reports that the students love doing meditation and after lunch come into the room and prepare. They also know the routine and don't like missing it. The benefits she reports are numerous. The students work right through the afternoon and are able to stay on task. It settles the more "boisterous" class members. It makes them calm, settled and able to concentrate. She reports that the students seem more organised for the afternoon activities. It also provides her with time to prepare and gain her thoughts, especially if she has had duty or meetings in the lunch break.

She reports that it normally takes students the whole of the term to get used to the process. Annette currently has some children in her class that are labelled with having "learning difficulties" including one child with ADHD. She reports that it is these students who benefit the most. One student in particular (whose parents were trying to have the student diagnosed with ADHD and placed on the drug Ritalin) responded very well to meditation and Annette's calm approach, so much so that other staff members had asked how she had been able to control him. He is currently not requiring Ritalin and told Annette that she had helped him to find "*the real me*".

Annette has seen no negative effects, in fact she reports that the relatively small amount of time spent meditating enables more learning to take place in the afternoon. She believes that many of the reasons that teachers don't teach meditation are centred on the lack of confidence teaching it. Many teachers don't know how to teach it and have difficulty with the time constraints in schools. She believes that people generally accept that meditation is beneficial and the term is more widely accepted. She feels that meditation should be offered across the whole school and much of it at present depends on the philosophy of the principal.

Experience 2 - Deborah

Deborah is an early childhood teacher of over 30 years experience who currently teaches a split class of Kindergarten/ Pre-primary. Deborah has been meditating for over 30 years and has taught it in the classroom for the whole duration of her career. Deborah teaches meditation every day following lunch. The meditation session lasts for approximately 15-20 minutes. She also uses meditation if her class are "*hanging from the ceiling*" at other times of the day to calm them down and restore focus.

Deborah has the full support of her principal and discussed teaching meditation with all parents at the beginning of the year during her parent-teacher introduction talk. She explained to the parents that the class would be doing meditation and the reasons why. No parents had any concerns or complaints.

Deborah presents meditation as something of great value to her class. She describes to the children that it is very important to do all aspects of school work but the best way to control their brain and to understand how it operates is by learning to meditate. She discusses problem solving and great listening skills with the children and how meditation helps with these areas. Deborah also discusses that they have a magic third eye in their mind that can help them greatly.

Deborah's class made their own set of "meditation manners" and she expresses that they really look forward to meditation time. She finds that the class is often able to do structured activities in the afternoon, which is normally not the case with this age-group. She explains that it normally takes the kindy children a few months to learn and uses activities such as drawing and painting to validate what they are doing as a follow-up when they first learn.

Deborah uses a combination of breathing, body awareness and visualization. She asks students to get their cushions and find comfortable positions. She often starts her meditation session with a song to get rid of any tension or excess energy. The children do some deep breathing and begin their visualization. Deborah discusses with the children that Meditation helps them to learn to "control their own bodies".

As an experienced meditation practitioner, Deborah often makes up her own visualizations to suit the children's needs on top of using meditations from a book or CD.

Deborah says that she finds children who have trouble controlling their behaviour seem to show the greatest improvement. She encourages all teachers to just try it and persevere and they will see the benefits for themselves. An incident she recalls from earlier this year to describe the above is when one of her more challenging students was asked a question and the student asked her to give him a moment. He stopped and shut his eyes, and said he was listening for the answer, which he then gave. Deborah recalls that in class they often discuss as part of meditation that *if you stop and are quiet for a few seconds, the answer may come to you*, this was confirmation for her.

Deborah reports that she has seen no negative effects nor has she had a negative reaction from parents. She believes that discussing it at the start of the year parent meeting prevents this from happening.

She also believes meditation supports social and emotional health and the values within schools. She supports teaching it as part of the curriculum but feels that to teach it you must value meditation and understand its benefits. Another teacher at her school who works through a series of year levels teaches meditation to all her classes and she has been asked by another male teacher at her school to come into his class and show him how it is done. There has been great interest generated by the success in her class.

The main barriers to introducing it into a school, says Deborah, are the fact that teachers don't know how to teach it and already feel they have an overburdened curriculum. She believes that if the research on its benefits is presented to teachers and that they can see that it is not hard to teach, more teachers would take it on.

These are the meditation manners that Deb's class came up with:
- *Stay still*
- *Be very quiet*
- *Close your eyes and engage your third eye*
- *Respect your friends*
- *Make your body floppy*
- *Close your fingers in the meditation position*

Experience 3 - Wendy

Wendy is the very resourceful teacher I mentioned in the paragraph on meditation aids earlier in the book. Wendy has been kind enough to share her classroom experience.

I have always done relaxation with the children in my classroom after lunch. I find that it is a fantastic way for children to wind down but at the same time revitalise their energy.

The children play a big part in setting up and putting away for relaxation time. The line leaders go into class first, the girl line leader gives out the mats and the boy line leader gives out the eye pillows. The rest of the children then come inside. They line up to get a mat first and if they want they get an eye pillow. The children then find a spot on the floor and then 'top and tail' this is to avoid children talking to each other. If the children want a blanket on them they put their hand up and I quickly put one on them. I have only started putting the blanket on the children this year, as a few of them asked for it. I have a Yoga teacher who always asks you if you want a blanket on and I must admit I do always have one while I am doing meditation. I then begin with the meditation/relaxation. Sometimes we just have music and other times I would put on a listening story or read a story to the children. Other times I would select a piece of music and then guide the children on an adventure. For example I used a piece of music from Tubular Bells 2 which sounded like space music and we went to a planet and met aliens.

I alternate the words relaxation and meditation with the children. It is also a great way for children to develop listening skills as well as their imaginations. In the beginning many children will copy what another child has said and then over the year they will develop their own imaginations. After the session, children fold and pack away their own blankets, mats and eye pillows. We then either draw what we saw on our adventure or discuss in class; some days we even do both. The children come up with some great illustrations of what they think the certain adventures look like.

Colour, Energy and Meditation

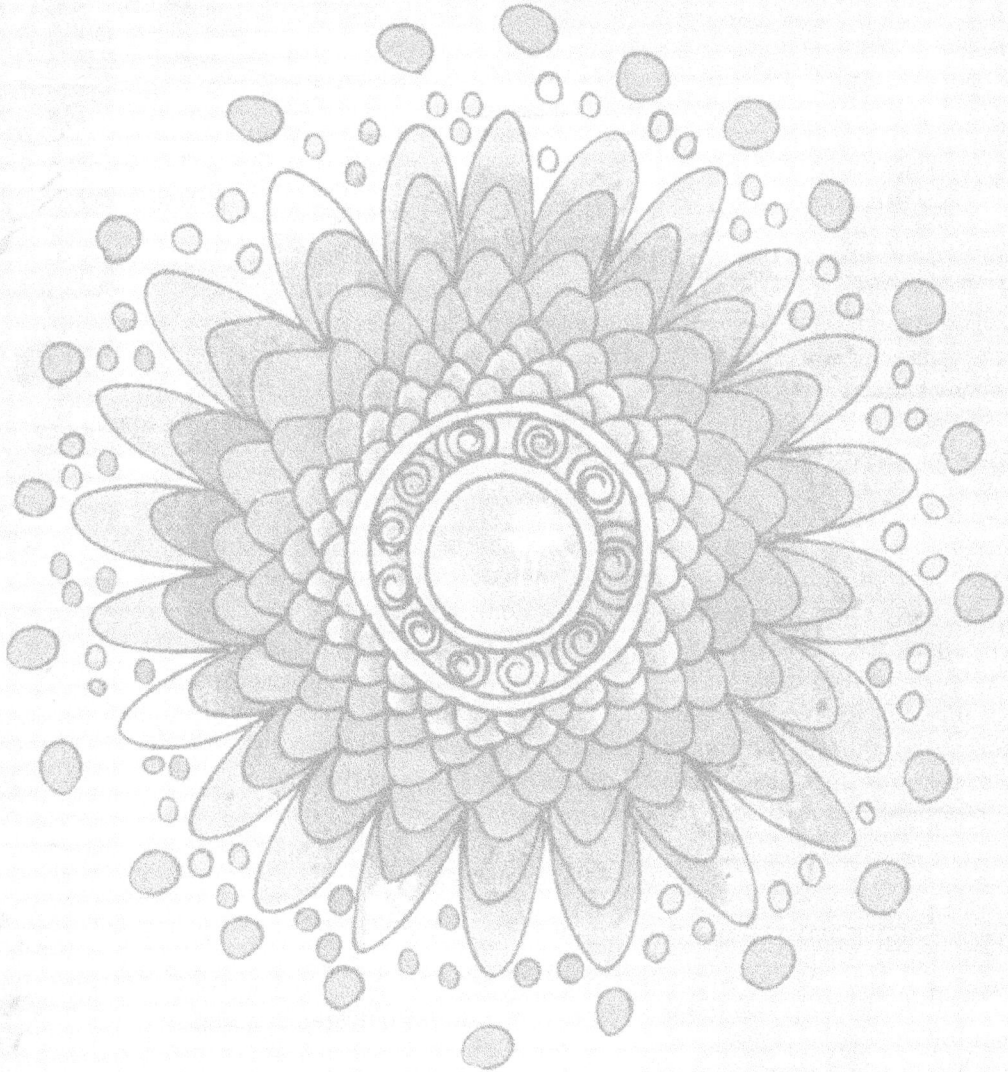

Colour, Energy and Meditation

Over the last decade there has been a huge increase in the number of people seeking complimentary medicine. Energy medicine has become a very popular modality for those seeking alternative treatments. Energy work proposes that imbalances in the body's energy field can lead to ill health and associated issues. The body's health can be restored by rebalancing the body through a variety of different healing methods. For the purposes of this book we are looking at how colour, energy and meditation can work together. Making children aware of their energy centres, the healing properties of colour and the meditation process and provides them with both the knowledge and the tools for balancing their bodies.

If this concept is too left of field for you, then by all means skip to the next chapter. For those who are interested in reading further, I have included a basic summary and a simple outline that is relevant to children and to those working with children.

We are all made of energy. Our physical body, our feelings, beliefs and thoughts all interact together to create an energy flow within our body. Our energy interacts with the people and the environment around us. Everything around us takes energy in and releases it. How often do you go to a busy shopping centre and come home exhausted and frazzled? This is our energy interacting with all the people, noise, lights and shops that surround us. However, if you go to an uncrowded beach and sit and relax by the ocean, you feel much more relaxed and calm. You only have yourself and the healing energy of nature to contend with. Although this energy is invisible to us we can feel its subtle affects on us.

The Chakra Energy System has its roots in the eastern hemisphere but is now widely accepted in western natural-healing modalities. There is sometimes an aura of mysticism surrounding the word "chakra" and the beliefs associated with this subtle energy system. It has been used for thousands of years by yogis and healers who believe that illness and disorders commonly first manifest themselves in the chakras. The word chakra comes from the Sanskrit term meaning "wheel" or "spin". In a nutshell, our body is made up of spinning vortexes of energy called chakras which are directly associated with the physical, emotional, mental and spiritual health of a person. Each chakra is also associated with specific organs, glands and body systems. The 7 major chakras are indicated on the diagram below and are aligned along the spinal column. All seven chakras resonate at their own specific frequency corresponding to one of the colours of the rainbow. They spin in a clockwise direction.

Chakras

In a healthy body the energy flow is harmonious and all the chakras are balanced and of a similar size. If our chakras are blocked or out of balance, the energy does not flow harmoniously. Chakras may be spinning too fast or too slow i.e. under active or over-active. They may be spinning the wrong way. Some may be larger than others or they may be blocked or congested. If a chakra is out of sync, it may eventually affect other neighbouring chakras and it is usually felt physically, mentally and emotionally. Imagine a machine with a series of wheels or cogs spinning. If one is going to fast or too slow then the whole machine will go out of balance and eventually stop working. Our body or machine will be physically imbalanced and we will end up with ill health.

When I discuss this with children I explain that everyone has a rainbow that is part of them and that it is

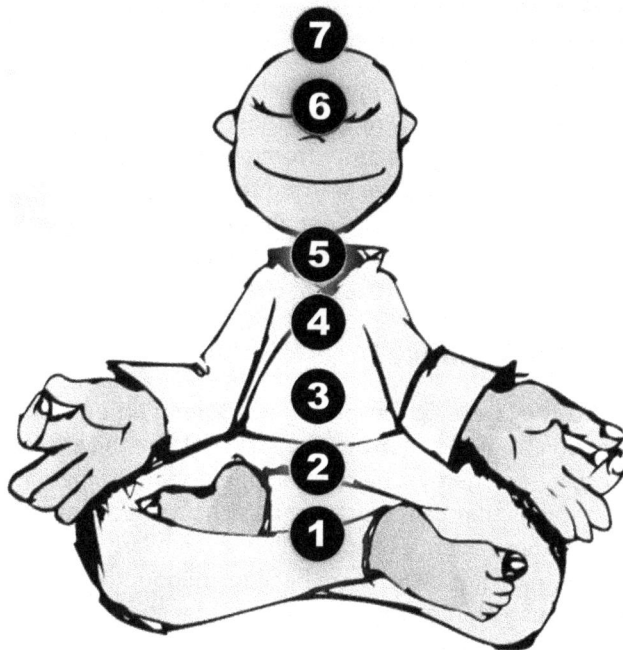

The 7 Major Chakras

1. Base or Root Chakra
Colour: Red
Location: Base of the spine

2. Sacral Chakra
Colour: Orange
Location: Just below the navel

3. Solar Plexus Chakra
Colour: Yellow
Location: Just above the navel

4. Heart Chakra
Colour: Green
Location: Centre of the chest, just above the heart

5. Throat Chakra
Colour: Blue
Location: In our throat

6. Brow or Third Eye Chakra
Colour: Indigo
Location: Centre of the forehead, between our eyebrows

7. Crown Chakra
Colour: Violet
Location: On top of our head

made up of 7 energy centres called "Chakras". I explain that blocked energy centres can lead to feeling out of balance, or stuck and can make them sick. If they keep their rainbow clear of any blockages they will always feel balanced and full of energy.

A child's chakras are always developing and throughout a child's life to adulthood they each become a focus for a period of time. For example, the root chakra is the most important in the early years as this is where children physically develop, get their sense of security from and develop the feeling of being grounded. The sacral chakras development is where emotions are starting to develop and so on. For ease of reading I have summarised the main focus of each chakra, its main functions and how it relates to a child when it is working and not working, in table format. You may be interested in the similarities with diagnosed disorders such as ADHD and Autism relating directly to issues with the root chakra, throat chakra and brow chakra.

How do Chakras get out of Balance?

Children are like big sponges as they develop, absorbing everything around them. The chakras are similar, drawing in energy and information from their surroundings. It could be the energy from a colour vibration or a radio wave or even another person's energy. Environments, emotions, experiences, feelings, thoughts and traumas are some of the main things that can affect a child's chakras and impede healthy energy flow. Our chakras are thought to store all of these energies and our chakras regularly need to be balanced or cleared out of any blockages. We often hear that adult issues stem back to childhood experiences. This can be likened to the energy from this experience being stored or stuck in a particular chakra. As an example, imagine a child is constantly bullied at school and told that they are fat and no good at anything. This upsets them and they start to absorb the emotions and words which can affect their self worth. This would affect their solar plexus chakra which governs confidence, self esteem and personal power.

Ways for Children to Balance their Chakras

Children can balance their chakras in a variety of ways. They may be not be aware they have an imbalance nor do they realise they are actually helping balance their bodies energy by doing some of the activities below. They are all self explanatory and are covered throughout the book. The ones I generally use with children include:

- Meditation
- Visualisation
- Calming Techniques
- Yoga
- Aromatherapy
- Colour
- Affirmations
- Exercise
- Positive Attitude
- Music/Sound
- Crystals

Many of the visualisations and exercises in this book ask children to use colour or identify any part of the body that is not feeling great. Children will intuitively go to the colour they require and will be constantly using techniques to create balance and harmony. Each section of visualisations corresponds to a chakra colour. All of the visualisations have affirmations associated with both the colour they represent and the specific visualisation.

The visualisations are constantly exploring a child's physical, mental, spiritual and emotional being. The rainbow visualisations are particularly good for balancing **all** the chakras. The beauty is that by learning the techniques in the book and participating in the visualisations, a child will be constantly balancing their energy centres.

When teaching meditation to children the root chakra is very important. Grounding a child helps them to stay calm and focused throughout the meditation. The suggested outline for meditation practice has a beginning journey and taking deep breaths to help ground a child and make them feel safe and secure. As mentioned previously, if you are not relaxed and calm as a teacher or parent doing meditation with your children, your energy will affect the experience. Make sure you are grounded before beginning.

I should mention that there are some beautiful music CD's available that are specifically for balancing the chakras. These can be played in the house or classroom as background music. I often play them when my children go to bed at night.

There are also sounds that children can make to balance their chakras and crystals they can wear or place under their pillows. For more detailed information on this and other aspects of the Chakra Energy System see the books below as suggested resources.

The Book of Chakra Healing: Liz Simpson - Gaia Books
Chakra Meditation: Swami Saradanandra - Duncan Baird Publishers

Chakra Colour	Function/Focus	Relation to child	If out of balance
Root or Base Chakra **RED**	**Physical Existence** Feeling grounded Feeling active and centred Survival instincts	Strength Fitness Health Security	Feel spacey Don't feel safe Depressed Can't focus/concentrate Excessive energy Obsessions Food & Health issues
Sacral Chakra **ORANGE**	**Emotions/Intimacy** Ability to accept others Ability to accept new experiences Ability to accept Oneself Sexuality	Creativity Happiness Being in control Joy Depth of feelings	Angry Fearful Rigid in their ways Can't accept change Emotional instability Allergies Tired
Solar Plexus Chakra **YELLOW**	**Power & Identity** Personal power In control of our lives	Self control Inner strength Vitality & Energy Confidence Self image	Fearful Stress & Anxiety Low self esteem Digestive issue Bullying Oversensitive
Heart Chakra **GREEN**	**Love & Relationships** Our ability to love and forgive Relationships	Harmony Balance Love & respect Friendship Empathy Compassion Self acceptance	Irrational Sad Lonely Anti-social Co-dependant Asthma
Throat Chakra **BLUE**	**Self Expression & Life Purpose** Our ability to communicate Creative connection	Self expression Honesty Communications Choosing right from wrong Courage Listening	Afraid to voice their opinion or too vocal Difficulty listening to others Lack of purpose Perfectionism
Brow Chakra (Third Eye) **INDIGO**	**Clear Perspective** Our ability to see the big picture Deals with senses Decision making	Intuition Peace of mind Meditation Wisdom & Study Imagination Negotiation Self reflection	Headaches Stress Lack of sleep Memory loss or forgetful Nightmares Sleep disorders Headaches
Crown Chakra **VIOLET**	**Connection** Our ability to feel connected Dreams, visions and hopes	Unity Feeling like they belong Inner and outer beauty Spirituality and awareness	Learning disabilities Over intellectual Depression Apathy Confusion Obsessive thinking Feel they don't fit in Feel misunderstood

VISUALISATIONS

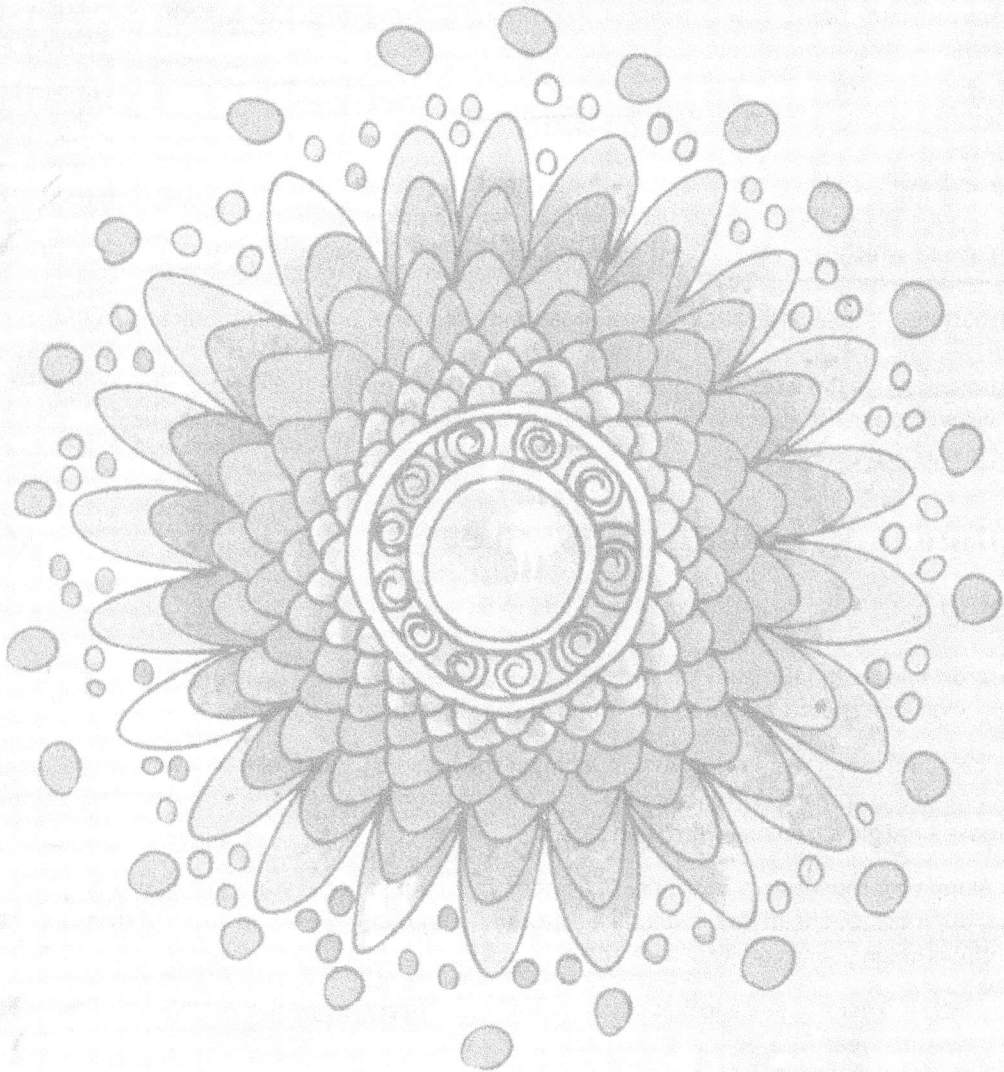

Points to Remember

- The visualisations in *Rainbow Dreaming* are separated under each colour of the rainbow and each section focuses on different key issues or values.
- You can randomly select a visualisation or work your way through the book.
- You may wish to choose your visualisation according to the affirmation or theme associated with it.
- *Italics* have been used for all spoken parts in the meditation to alert the reader and to enable the meditation to flow.
- Remember to pause between each paragraph or at open ended questions to allow the child time to process.
- You can leave the children in the open-ended finish of the visualisation as long as you like i.e. *Spend as long as you like enjoying the fresh sea air...* It will depend on your class or child.
- You can use whichever version of the beginning or ending sequence that you wish or you can use your own.
- Affirmations are included with each visualisation to reinforce positive self talk and to provide a point of focus.
- Each visualisation has a set of rainbow thoughts to prompt further discussion or to use in a sharing circle.
- The visualisations listed under the **Rainbow** section tend to be slightly longer and focus predominantly on achieving balance.

Beginning and Ending Sequences

Beginning

Find a comfortable position, close your eyes and be very, very still. Breathe in and out, in through your nose and out through your mouth. Listen to the sound of your breath for a moment.

You see a beautiful moonbeam of white light coming towards you. You feel the moonbeam as it reaches the top of your head and spreads down your whole body right to your toes. The white light completely surrounds you and makes you glow. You feel warm and safe.

You walk along your moonbeam and there in front of you, hanging on a star is a big blue hat. This is a Magic Worry hat, put it on your head and it will take away anything that is worrying you and that busy feeling that you sometimes get in your mind. You place the hat back on the star and feel calm and quiet.

You walk a little further and see another star. It has a beautiful crystal pendant hanging on it. This is a magic pendant for you to wear. This pendant will protect you while you go on your special journey. You place the pendant around your neck.

Just relax and enjoy the ride as your moonbeam takes you to a special place to start your magical adventure.

Imagine...

Shortened Beginning

Find a comfortable position, close your eyes and be very, very still. Breathe in and out. Listen to the sound of your breath for a moment.

You see a beautiful moonbeam of white light coming towards you, the white light surrounds you and you feel warm and safe.

You walk along the moonbeam to the Magic Worry Hat. You put it on, let go of all your worries and hang it back on the star.

You continue walking to the crystal pendant. You place it around your neck. This pendant will protect while you go on your special journey.

Just relax and enjoy the ride as your moonbeam takes you to a special place to start your magical adventure.

Imagine...

Alternative Beginning

Find a comfortable position, close your eyes and be very, very still.

Breathe in and out, listen to the sound of your breath for a few moments... Feel your body relaxing, feel the tension leave.

Continue to take some deep breaths, on each exhale imagine all your worries are leaving your body.

You feel very safe and very relaxed as your imagination takes you on a special journey.

Imagine...

Ending

When you are ready, step back onto your moonbeam. Place the crystal pendant back on the star.

Keep walking until you pass the Worry Hat and you are back where you started from.

Thank your moonbeam for a great adventure.

Wiggle your fingers and toes, stretch out as far as you can and slowly open your eyes.

Repeat the Affirmation

Alternative Ending

When you are ready, wiggle your fingers and toes, stretch out as far as you can and slowly open your eyes.

Repeat the Affirmation

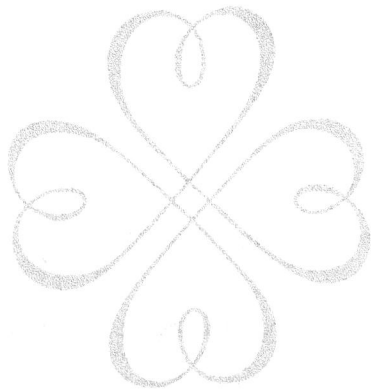

RED

Red is an energising colour. Red is the colour of strength and courage. Red helps us feel safe and secure.

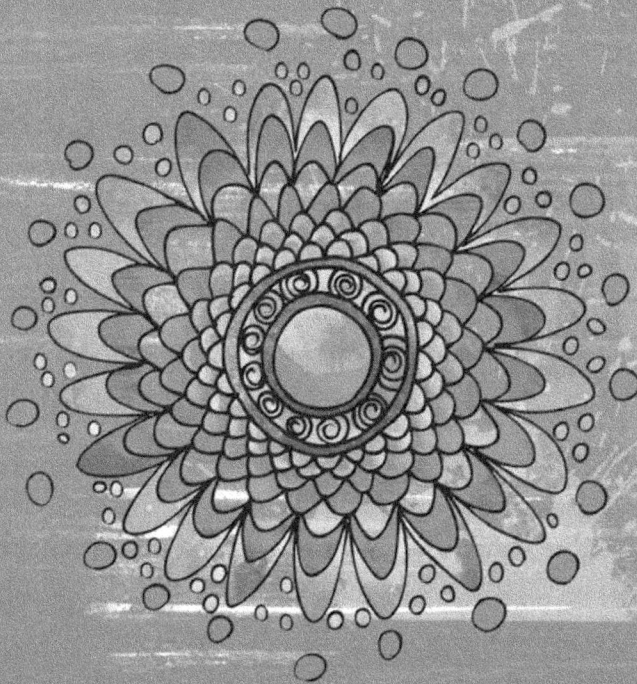

Red Affirmations

I am safe

I am healthy

I am strong

I am responsible

I am powerful

I am secure

I deserve the best

I love the earth

I make healthy choices and
take care of my body

I enjoy the colour red

Red

Imagine that you are sitting on a comfortable chair in the centre of a room. This room is a special room, because when you say a colour, the whole room turns that colour. Today your colour is red.

You say the word red and watch as the room now turns completely red. First the walls turn red, then the ceiling, the floor, even the chair you are sitting on. It is as if the whole room is bathed in red light. Take a moment to look around the room. What else do you see? Put your hand into the red light. What does the colour red feel like?

You take a deep breath in through your nose and then let it go out through your mouth. You count in two, three, and four and out two, three, and four. As you breathe in imagine that the colour red is coming up from the floor of the room through the bottom of your feet. Every time you take a breath in, the colour spreads further up through your body. It is as if you are breathing in the colour red. What does the colour red smell like?

The colour spreads from the tips of your toes, up your legs, over your hips and stomach, up your chest, over your arms and fingers, up through your neck and shoulders, over your face until it reaches the top of your head and you are completely red. How does the colour red make you feel? What thoughts or ideas come to you when you are the colour red?

Spend as long as you like enjoying the colour red...

I enjoy
the colour
red

Rainbow Thoughts

- *Colour can be used to help balance our body's energy.*

- *Red is a powerful colour that can give us courage or strength when we need it.*

- *Red is a good colour to wear or think about if you are feeling unsettled or a bit spacey.*

- *Red is a good colour to wear when you are going somewhere new as it is the colour of strength and courage.*

Magic Garden

Imagine that you are standing next to a large golden gate. Can you see its shiny handle? This gate is the entrance to a very special place. It is the entrance to your own magic garden. Only you can enter the garden. The gate will not open for anyone else. You touch the gate and walk inside. As soon as you enter your garden you feel calm and relaxed. All the stress and tension leaves your body and you feel very, very safe.

You notice a basket in front of you. It is full of seeds. These are magic seeds and you can create whatever you wish in your garden. These seeds don't need water. They only need your positive thoughts and creativity. Your positive thoughts are so powerful they can make anything grow. Spend time planting your seeds and watch as they grow and bloom around you.

Look around your garden at all the wonderful things you have created. What do you see? Can you see the beautiful green trees? Everything in your garden is so radiant. There are so many colours and so much to explore. You walk around your garden. What plants and flowers can you see? You stop and gently touch them. What do they feel like? Can you smell the sweet perfume in the air? What else can you smell? Notice what is under your feet. Is it soft green grass or something else? Look at the colour of the sky? Are there any clouds?

Now you have created such a magical garden, think about the wonderful things your garden has attracted to it. Are there any butterflies or beetles? Perhaps there are some earthworms. Do you have any magical creatures living in your garden?

Spend time listening to the sounds in your garden. What can you hear? Can you hear the sound of birds twittering or perhaps the sound of trickling water? Is there a pond? What else can you hear in your garden?

As you continue to explore your garden, see if you can find a special place where you can relax? Perhaps there is a hammock or a big comfy lounge under the tree. This special place is there for you to relax and enjoy some time on your own, solve a problem or just think quietly. When you find it, lie down and take some deep breaths.

While you are relaxing in your special place a little bird lands on your shoulder. The bird whispers a special message in your ear. This message is something you need to know to help you in your life. You listen very carefully. What does the little bird tell you? You thank the little bird and watch as it flies off.

Spend as long as you like relaxing in your Magic Garden. You can visit your magic garden whenever you wish, all you have to do is open the golden gate and enter...

I always have my own safe, quiet place inside me

Rainbow Thoughts

- *When we are feeling stressed, tired or confused it helps to find a quiet space to take some deep breaths and relax.*

- *Our thoughts are so important. If you think positive, loving thoughts you will help the garden inside of you to grow.*

- *Sometimes answers come to us when we take the time to listen quietly.*

- *You can create your own safe place in your mind and visit it whenever you need to.*

Peaceful Warrior

Imagine that you are standing in front of a big golden throne in the heart of a grand palace. The throne is made of thick red velvet and covered in hundreds of sparkling jewels. It is the most beautiful throne you have ever seen. Sitting in the throne is a great King. The King is a big strong man. His eyes are very kind and you feel very safe standing in front of him. The King has invited you here today to present you with two very special gifts.

The King hands you your first gift. It is a large shield. You take the shield into your hands. It is so light it feels like you have a feather in your hand. What does your shield look like? What do you think it is made from? The King tells you that this is no ordinary shield, it is a magic shield. This shield is always there to protect you. The King explains to you that the shield can help you when someone is not being kind towards you or perhaps saying things that make you feel upset or angry. Only happy, kind thoughts and feelings will pass through this shield, anything else will bounce off and become dust. You thank the King and clip your magic shield onto your back.

The King now tells you that your second gift has arrived. You feel a presence to the right of you and turn to find your own guardian animal. Can you see it? What type of animal is it? Your guardian animal can only be seen by you and is always there to help you and protect you. Your guardian animal is very wise and is able to help you answer questions. You touch your animal. What does it feel like? It tells you its name. Can you hear it? You feel strong and protected with your guardian by your side.

The King tells you that you are now a peaceful warrior, armed with your magic shield and guardian animal. Whenever you need your shield and animal, you can call to them and they will appear. You thank the King.

You spend some time in the palace gardens getting to know your guardian animal and practising using your shield. When you are ready, walk out through the palace gates to begin a new adventure...

I am
safe
and protected

Rainbow Thoughts

- *We are equipped with many abilities inside us that act like a magic shield. We just need to learn how to tap into them.*

- *Sometimes people say things that make us upset or angry. Don't let these words change how you feel. Simply let them bounce off you and think of something that makes you feel strong and happy again.*

- *Our animal guide can help us tap into our inner wisdom and make us feel safe.*

Energy Bath

Imagine that you are sitting in a big bathtub. The bath is half full and you watch as it slowly fills up all around you. The water is so warm and it is making you feel very relaxed and calm. You notice a bottle of bubble bath on the side of the bath. You take off the cap and add some to the running water. You watch as the colour red swirls in the water. Before long the bath has turned completely red. There is a beautiful fresh fragrance which smells like strawberries, coming from the bath. Once the bath is full, you stretch out and lie back until water completely covers you and only your neck and head are showing. You feel very safe and secure lying in your red bubble bath.

You watch as the bubbles pop and fizz around you, tickling your neck as they move around. You notice that your toes are starting to tingle softly. It is a nice feeling and it slowly spreads up your feet to your knees and then up your legs. You feel your hips tingle, your stomach and your back. You are enjoying it so much that you find yourself giggling. The tingle starts in your fingers and moves to your hands, arms and all the way up your chest to your neck. Your whole body is now tingling and it feels like all your cells are being energised. All your aches and pains go away and any worries you have seem to dissolve with the bubbles. You feel fantastic.

As you soak in your energising bath you think about your body. Think about the things you could do to keep your body in good shape and feeling energised. Think about the sort of foods that you could eat or drink. What exercise you could do to keep your body fit?

Spend as long as you like soaking in your energy bath. When you are ready, get out of the bath, have a big stretch and feel how refreshed and energised you are. Come back and have an energy bath any time you need to...

I am

energised

Rainbow Thoughts

- *If you are feeling "fuzzy" in the head or low in energy try taking some deep breaths for a few minutes.*

- *Sometimes you feel like you don't have enough energy.
  This can be because we have too much happening in our life or we are stressed.*

- *Bubble baths, imaginary or real, are a great way to relax and re-energise.*

- *Exercise and fresh air is good for balancing energy and reenergising the body.*

Magic Carpet

Imagine that you are sitting on a magic carpet. It is has been woven with many beautiful richly coloured threads and edged with big gold tassels. Can you see any patterns on your carpet? What colours is your magic carpet made of? What does your carpet feel like to touch? You say the following magic words, I am free I am free I am free. You feel the carpet start to move as it slowly rises into the air with you on it. Even though it is a piece of carpet, it feels very strong and you feel very safe sitting on it. Today your magic carpet is going to take you on a ride to see some of the most amazing places in the world.

You feel the magic carpet start to rise a little higher. It is a wonderful feeling. You feel like you are floating above the ground. The carpet goes a little higher. You feel very relaxed. It seems the higher you go, the lighter you feel. Now your carpet starts to move forward. It moves very slowly at first then it starts to go a little faster. You start to smile and laugh because you feel very happy. It feels fantastic to be moving through the air on your carpet. The wind gently tickles your face. Your hair is blowing back in the breeze and you have not a care in the world. You move up a little higher into the clouds. Your magic carpets floats so that you can touch the clouds with your hands. What do they feel like? Do they feel soft and fluffy? What else can you see up on your magic carpet?

Now that you are used to travelling on your Magic carpet, it waits for you to tell it what to do. You are the master of the magic carpet, you can control how high it goes, how fast it goes and where you would like it to take you. All you have to do is say it in your mind. Say fast and feel your carpet speed up. Say slow and feel your carpet slow right down and gently drift along. Say up and feel it rise higher and higher. Now say down and feel it start to lower. You can do all sorts of amazing things on your carpet. Hold on to the sides and you can try zigging and zagging. You can sweep and dive through the air. It is so much fun riding on your magic carpet.

Now think about where you would like to visit and your carpet will take you there. Perhaps you would like to see another country and try some of its delicious food. Perhaps you would like to go high up into the mountains and see if you can find snow. You can visit all the oceans of the world, the African savannah or the rainforests and jungles. Perhaps you would like to see the great pyramids, or watch the whales and penguins frolic in the Arctic. There are so many choices. Sit quietly for a few moments and make your decision. When you are ready, say your destination and you are off.

Make sure you remember what you have seen so that you can tell your friends and family.

Spend as long as you like feeling light and free, enjoying the wonderful adventures your magic carpet takes you on. When you are ready, say the word home and it will bring you back to where you started...

I am free to make my own choices

Rainbow Thoughts

- *In our imagination we are free to go anywhere we wish.*

- *Sometimes when we have so many choices our mind gets jumbled and it is hard to make a decision. Spend a few moments relaxing and taking some deep breaths. This will help you with your choice.*

- *There are no limits to what we can create with our imagination.*

ORANGE

Orange is a fun and upifting colour. Orange is the colour of creativity and happiness. Orange helps us to understand our feelings.

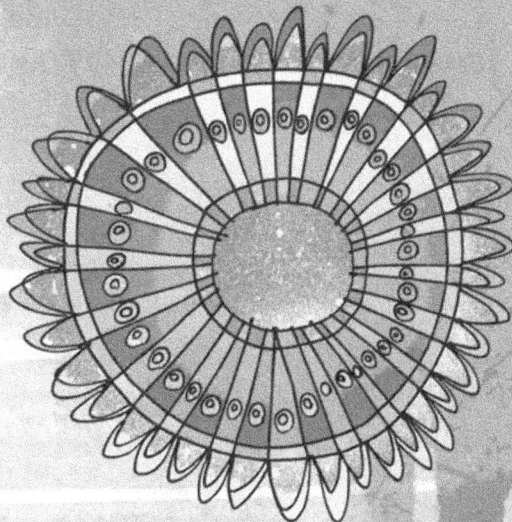

Orange Affirmations

I am creative

I am happy

I am worthy

I enjoy having fun

I am special

I enjoy my life

I am full of great ideas

I always have everything I need

I enjoy the colour orange

Orange

Imagine that you are sitting on a comfortable chair in the centre of a room. This room is a special room. When you say a colour, the whole room turns that colour. Today your colour is orange.

You say the word *orange* and watch as the room now turns completely orange. First the walls turn orange, then the ceiling, the floor, even the chair you are sitting on. It is as if the whole room is bathed in orange light. Take a moment to look around the room. What else do you see? Put your hand into the orange light. What does the colour orange feel like?

You take a deep breath in through your nose and then let it go out through your mouth. You count in two, three, and four and out two, three, and four. As you breathe in imagine that the colour orange is coming up from the floor of the room through the bottom of your feet. Every time you take a breath in, the colour spreads further up through your body. It is as if you are breathing in the colour orange. What does the colour orange smell like?

The colour spreads from the tips of your toes, up your legs, over your hips and stomach, up your chest, over your arms and fingers, up through your neck and shoulders, over your face until it reaches the top of your head and you are completely orange. How does the colour orange make you feel? What thoughts or ideas come to you when you are the colour orange?

Spend as long as you like enjoying the colour orange...

I enjoy

the colour

orange

Rainbow Thoughts

- *Colour can be used to help change our moods.*

- *Orange is a dynamic colour that helps to think of new ideas.*

- *Orange is a stimulating colour and helps with creativity.*

- *Orange is a fun colour. It is the colour of joy and happiness.*

Hot Air Balloon

Imagine that you are standing in a big field of lush green grass. It is a beautiful sunny day and there is a light breeze blowing. The breeze blows gently through your hair and you feel it soothing your face. You take in a deep breath and let the fresh air fill your lungs. You look around the field and see a hot air balloon in the distance. You walk towards it.

You watch as the giant balloon sways in the breeze. Can you see what colour the giant balloon is? You reach the basket and climb inside. The basket is very strong and sturdy and you feel very safe inside it. There is a comfortable seat for you to sit down on.

Now think about all the things that make you feel happy. It can be a place, person, animal, your favourite pastime or hobby, your favourite food, anything that makes you feel happy. As you think about the things that make you feel happy, the balloon gently rises. It seems happy thoughts help to power this hot air balloon. Keep thinking happy thoughts and watch as the balloon gently lifts in the air.

If any thought comes and makes you feel sad or angry, imagine yourself tossing it out of the balloon basket to be carried away by the breeze. Throw any negative thoughts out as well and imagine them floating away. All your worries seem to disappear as you move higher into the air. You feel very light and free and your mind feels clear. You feel very safe and secure because your balloon will always stay afloat and will only go as high as you wish it to.

Your balloon now starts moving across the blue sky and over the landscape below. Now take the time to look out at your surroundings. Can you see the white fluffy clouds? Can you feel the cool breeze blowing on your face? It is so peaceful being up in the air as you gently drift over houses, trees, parks ...

What else can you see below? Can you see the birds? Can you see the hills in the distance?

You continue to sail the skies in your hot air balloon. Perhaps you can watch the sunset while up in your balloon and see the sky change into beautiful shades of purple, pink and blue. Maybe you will cross an ocean and watch the sea creatures swimming below.

Spend as long as you like enjoying the ride in your hot air balloon and thinking lots of happy thoughts. When you are ready simply say the words *back to the field* and your balloon with return you to the lush green field you started in. You can come back and go for a balloon ride any time you wish....

I choose

happiness

Rainbow Thoughts

- *You can choose how you wish to start each day.*

- *How often do you hear people say "I woke up grumpy" or "I woke up on the wrong side of the bed"? There is no reason to stay grumpy for the rest of the day.*

- *Think of things that make you happy and this will make you feel good. This will help to set your mood and thought patterns for the day.*

Magic Easel

Imagine that you are standing in a beautiful white room. The room has beautiful big windows that are covered with soft, sheer, white curtains. You watch as the breeze gently moves the curtains in and out. It almost looks like the curtains are breathing. You look around and see that the floorboards are also painted white. It is very refreshing and peaceful standing in this beautiful white room. You take a deep breath. The air smells clean and fresh.

You notice that standing right in the middle of the room there is a giant white canvas. It is the only item in your white room. Your canvas is resting on a beautiful golden art easel. You move towards it to take a closer look. The easel looks as if it is made of solid gold. It glistens and sparkles. You run your hands over its surface. What does it feel like? It tells you that it is a special magic easel and anything you picture in your mind will automatically appear on the canvas as a colourful picture.

You try something simple to start with. Perhaps you imagine a flower, or a leaf. Watch as this picture magically appears on the canvas. Now try imagining your closest friend or a pet and watch them magically appear. If you make a mistake you can easily rub it out by waving your hand. The easel tells you that mistakes are okay and they help you to learn. You can make as many as you want.

Now think of all the things you have to be grateful for in your life. It can be things such as the home you live in, fresh running water in your tap, the food you have to eat each day, friends, family, pets, your health, toys, games, sport, art. You watch as they appear one after the other on your special easel and canvas.

Now think about one thing that you are really grateful for today and watch it magically appear on your canvas. What can you see? What colours appear on your canvas? How does it make you feel? There are so many things to think about. Sometimes it is easy to forget how many things there are to be grateful for.

Spend as long as you like drawing on your magic easel. Come back and visit any time you wish to think about all the wonderful things that you are surrounded by each and every day...

I have everything I need

Rainbow Thoughts

- *Sometimes it is good to sit and think about all the things you have instead of worrying about what you don't have.*

- *You may realise that you actually have everything you need already but have not taken the time to notice.*

- *Noticing simple pleasures and acknowledging the things you have in life makes you feel happier.*

- *Making mistakes is part of life. It helps us to learn. It is better to have made a mistake than to have not tried at all.*

- *Mistakes can be the stepping stones to success!*

Bridge to Happiness

Imagine that you are standing in a park. It is a beautiful sunny day. You can see white fluffy clouds drifting across the blue sky. You are surrounded by tall trees and lush green grass. You take a deep breath. What can you smell? You listen carefully to the sounds in the park. Can you hear any birds chirping or perhaps you hear the sound of laughter as children run and play in the park?

In the distance you see a bridge. It is made of stone and wood and sits across a stream that runs through the park. You walk towards the bridge. You notice the water gently gurgling and moving its way downstream. The sound of the water running is very calming and peaceful.

You step up to walk across the bridge and notice that there is a big bin next to the entrance. This bin is a magical bin. It wants you to put anything in it that makes you unhappy or sad. You won't be able to walk across the bridge until you have let go of these things. Take a few deep breaths and think about what makes you feel sad, unhappy or out of sorts. It may be something that upsets you or a fear you have. Imagine letting it go and throwing it into the bin. It doesn't matter how many things there are, just keep throwing them in the bin until you feel better.

Once you have finished letting go, you can step up onto the bridge. Take a deep breath in and start to walk across the bridge. You feel light and free. The further you walk the better you feel. As you walk across the bridge think of all the things that make you happy. It could be your family, a friend, a pet, an activity, anything at all that makes you happy.

Keep thinking about what makes you happy and feel yourself start to smile. Your energy levels start to pick up and soon you are running across the bridge to get to the other side. Once you reach the other side of the bridge you feel a huge smile light up your face. In front of you are all the things that make you happy. They are here for you to enjoy. It is such a good feeling to be happy.

Spend as long as you like smiling, laughing and feeling the joy of being happy. Remember you can come back and cross the bridge to happiness anytime you wish...

I choose
to be happy

Rainbow Thoughts

- *Happiness comes from within. Don't rely on other people or things to make you happy.*

- *Find out what makes you laugh and makes you happy, then do those things more often.*

- *One of the best ways to make you feel better is to smile and to think happy thoughts.*

Reflection Pool

Imagine that you are standing in a rainforest. You are surrounded by tall trees and lush vegetation. It is a nice sunny day and you can feel a very gentle breeze brush across your face. You watch the sunlight as it peaks through the forest canopy and makes a pattern on the forest floor. There are vines twisting up tree trunks and ferns and flowers. What else do you see?

You take a deep breath in and fill your lungs with the fresh forest air and take in the aromas of the rainforest. What do you smell? Do any of the flowers growing have a perfume to them?

You start to walk through the rainforest. It is very peaceful and you feel very safe. You listen carefully. What do you hear? Perhaps you hear the sounds of birds as they weave and dive through the trees or call to each other. Do you hear any crickets?

You hear the sound of water running in the distance? You decide to follow the sound and find a small stream winding its way over pebbles and rocks. You walk along the stream until you come to a beautiful big pool of water. The pool of water is very still and clear. You can see the pebbles on the bottom. You sit down next to the pond and enjoy the quiet.

As you are looking at the pool you realise that you can see your reflection. The pool is so clean and clear it almost looks like a mirror. You look closely and realise that your reflection in the pond is smiling and full of joy. Your reflection waves to you and you wave back. Your reflection seems very happy and excited to see you.

Your reflection then shows you surrounded by a big glittering star and points to you. It is telling you that you are a shining star. Then it shows you a big number 1. It is telling you that you are number 1 and to believe in yourself at all times. Now it shows you a big love heart. What do you think it is trying to tell you? Watch carefully as your reflection sends you some more messages. What do they say?

The reflection shows you a final message *I am worthy*. It asks you to say it three times every day. You repeat *I am worthy, I am worthy, I am worthy*. You are really enjoying your time at the reflection pool. Your confidence seems to grow the more time you spend there. It is a great feeling. You feel happy and content.

Spend as long as you like at the reflection pool enjoying your own company and what your reflection in showing you. You can come back anytime you wish...

ı enjoy learning
more about
myself

Rainbow Thoughts

- *Sometimes we need to spend some time alone to be totally comfortable with ourselves and to get to know ourselves better.*

- *If you are not feeling confident, try talking to yourself in the mirror. Use some positive affirmations to make you feel more self assured.*

- *Sometimes we have to remember to love ourselves.*

- *People who feel worthy are happier and less stressed than those people who don't feel good about themselves.*

YELLOW

Yellow is a **thinking** colour.
Yellow is the colour of
inner strength
and **confidence.**
Yellow helps us to
learn.

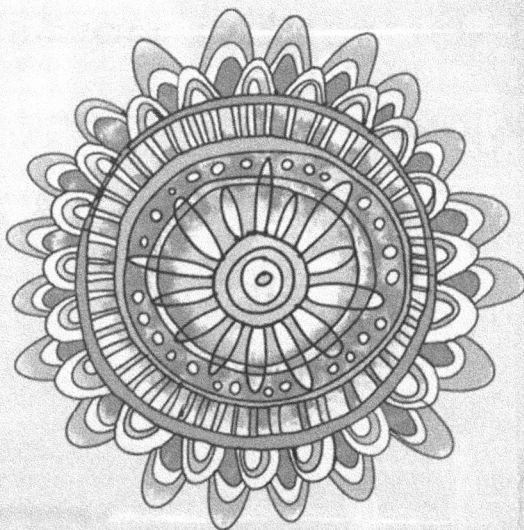

Yellow Affirmations

I am valuable

I am confident

I think positive thoughts

I respect myself

I have potential

I enjoy learning

I deserve good things

I am brave

I use positive words

I enjoy the colour yellow

Yellow

Imagine that you are sitting on a comfortable chair in the centre of a room. This room is a special room. When you say a colour, the whole room turns that colour. Today your colour is yellow. You say the word *yellow* and watch as the room now turns completely yellow. First the walls turn yellow, then the ceiling, the floor, even the chair you are sitting on. It is as if the whole room is bathed in warm yellow sunlight. Take a moment to look around the room. What else do you see? Put your hand into the yellow light. What does the colour yellow feel like?

You take a deep breath in through your nose, and then let it go out through your mouth. You count in two, three, and four and out two, three, and four. As you breathe in, imagine that the colour yellow is coming up from the floor of the room through the bottom of your feet. Every time you take a breath in the colour spreads further up through your body. It is as if you are breathing in the colour yellow. What does the colour yellow smell like?

The colour spreads from the tips of your toes, up your legs, over your hips and stomach, up your chest, over your arms and fingers, up through your neck and shoulders, over your face until it reaches the top of your head and you are completely yellow. How does the colour yellow make you feel? What thoughts or ideas come to you when you are the colour yellow?

Spend as long as you like enjoying the colour yellow...

I enjoy

the colour

yellow

Rainbow Thoughts

- *Colour can be used to help re-energise our body.*

- *Yellow is a warm colour that radiates joy.*

- *Yellow helps us to feel better about ourselves and helps to increase our confidence.*

- *Yellow is a good colour to have around you when you want to study or learn something new.*

Beanstalk

Imagine that you are standing in your magic garden. You look down towards your hand and see that you are holding a magic bean. You plant the bean in the ground and water it with your watering can. You watch the ground and see a little green shoot coming out of the soil. It gets bigger and bigger and bigger until it gets so big and tall that it has reached high up into the clouds.

You decide to climb your beanstalk and see what is at the top. You start to climb up the beanstalk. The leaves feel soft but very strong. You feel quite safe as you climb higher and higher. You look down and see your garden getting smaller and smaller. What else do you see?

You keep climbing your beanstalk until you reach the clouds. It is so quiet and peaceful up in the clouds. The clouds are so soft and fluffy. They tickle your nose and face as you climb through them. It is so quiet and peaceful up in the clouds.

You climb through the clouds and see that your beanstalk has led you to a magical castle. It is a gigantic castle. Whoever lives here must be very tall. You walk towards the castle and see a sign. It says: *The Giant's Vegetable Garden. Please come in and visit.*

You look beyond the sign and see the biggest vegetables you have ever seen. There are gigantic carrots, broccoli, potatoes, lettuce and spring onions. They tower over you? You keep walking. What else can you see? What can you hear and smell?

All of a sudden a giant rabbit comes hopping towards you. Can you see him? The rabbit tells you that he takes care of the giant's garden. The rabbit tells you that a giant's garden shows how happy a giant is. If a giant's garden is healthy and all the vegetables are growing big and strong, it means the giant is happy. When the giant is sad, his garden does not grow very well. Soon the leaves droop and the vegetables wilt and disappear.

You ask the rabbit how the giant stays happy. The rabbit tells you that the giant's garden grows with positive words and positive thoughts, which makes him very happy. The rabbit tells you that for people like you who live at the bottom of the beanstalk, your garden of happiness lies inside you. If your garden is growing well you will feel healthy and balanced. If it is not growing well you feel sad and unwell.

You thank the rabbit for telling you his wonderful story and head back to your beanstalk. You climb back down through the clouds, down, down until you reach the ground.

Spend time relaxing and thinking about the positive thoughts and words you will use today to help your garden to grow...

Today I will think positive thoughts and use positive words

Rainbow Thoughts

- *Positive thoughts and positive words help to create positive experiences.*

- *Positive self-talk helps to develop positive attitudes.*

- *If we feel happy and positive in our mind then our body will reflect this.*

- *Try and start each day with a positive thought.*

Jungle Walk

Imagine that you are in a jungle. The air is warm, steamy and moist. You take a deep breath in and let your lungs fill with this moist jungle air. What does the jungle smell like? You look around and see the trunks of giant jungle trees that seem to reach up into the sky. Can you see the rays of sunlight peeking through and dappling their light on the wet shiny leaves? You reach out to touch them. How to they feel? There are lush ferns and creepers and vines that wrap gently around them. Some of the creepers have grown right up the tree trunks into the jungle canopy. What else can you see?

You look down to the floor of the jungle. It is covered in leaves and sticks and it feels quite soft to walk on. You look a little closer and see that the jungle floor is teeming with life. Can you see all the tiny insects crawling? Can you see the little family of red beetles walking along the giant fern leaves? Can you see the long, skinny worms wriggling along on top of the soft moist earth? What else do you see? Can you see the beautiful butterflies dancing from flower to flower? All the insects and creatures seem to be busily going about their day.

You decide to take a walk through the jungle to see what else you can find. You can make out a path and decide to follow. A friendly toucan flies down to meet you. Can you see its big beak and brightly coloured feathers? The toucan tells you there is no need to be afraid; you are safe in the jungle because everyone here is a friend. What other birds can you see? Can you see the small brown birds flitting from leaf to leaf?

You walk a little further and see a huge snake hanging from a tree. The snake is the most beautiful shades of yellow and green. The snake's body has patterns on it. Can you see the diamond shapes? What other patterns can you see? The snake seems to be smiling at you. You reach out to pat the snake. The snake feels smooth and slimy and is enjoying you patting him. Perhaps you want to ask the snake some questions about life in the jungle.

You hear some loud noises that sound like monkeys whooping. You watch as they swing through the jungle towards you. They land on the branch next to the snake and give him a big pat on the back. A little monkey swings off the branch and lands on your shoulder. He is soft and fluffy and his fur has many different shades of brown. Can you see the black and white monkeys waving to you from the very top of the tree?

You say goodbye to the snake and continue along your path. Your monkey friends follow overhead. What other jungle animals do you see as you follow the path? What colours and shapes are they? What noises do they make? Perhaps you can hear the crickets singing?

You pass through more shrubs and vines until you come to a clearing in the jungle. There, sitting in the middle is a beautiful tiger. The monkeys tell you not to be afraid because she is a friendly tiger. You walk towards the tiger. She has beautiful black stripes and her fur is orange and white. You reach out to touch her. What does it feel like? The tiger tells you she likes meeting people and making new friends.

The tiger tells you that everything that lives in the jungle comes in different shapes, colours and sizes. Some walk, some climb, some fly, some slither and some run, some have feathers, some have fur and others have scaly skin. There are big animals and little animals. There are crawling insects and flying insects. It makes the jungle more interesting. Imagine if there were only tigers in the jungle or only snakes. The tiger asks you to imagine a jungle without the sound of birds chirping and monkeys whooping? You continue to walk with the tiger meeting lots of new friends and taking in all the sights and sounds.

Spend as long as you like in the jungle and think about how wonderful our world is with all the different types of living things...

It's ok to be different

Rainbow Thoughts

- *Variety makes our world interesting*
- *Just like the creatures in the jungle, people come in all different shapes, sizes and colours*
- *Everyone is special and unique*
- *Think about what makes you special and unique*

The Worry Tree

Imagine that you are standing in a garden. It is a warm sunny day and the sky is clear and blue. There is a gentle breeze blowing and you feel it as it gently tickles your face. You take a big breath in and let the fresh clean air fill your lungs. You feel safe in this beautiful garden.

Now take a look around the garden. What do you see? Do you see any flowers? What colours are they? What else do you see growing in the garden? Can you see the lush green lawn or perhaps you can see birds or butterflies? You take a deep breath in. The air is fresh and clean and as it slowly fills your lungs you feel calm and relaxed. Perhaps you can also smell some of the beautiful perfumes coming from the flowers. What sounds can you hear in the garden?

Something catches your attention in the corner of the garden. It is beautiful big tree. The tree is very tall and it looks like it has been in the garden for a very long time. It has a thick trunk and its branches are covered in lush green leaves. You move closer and touch it with your hand. You feel a tingle in your hand. There is something very special about this tree. The tree tells you that it is a Worry Tree. It tells you to sit down against its trunk and it will take all your worries away.

You sit down and relax against the tree. It feels cool against your back and you can feel your back start to tingle. It is a nice feeling. The leaves shade you and you feel very safe. Your tree tells you to take some deep breaths and tell it about anything that is worrying you. It might be something that has upset you or makes you feel unhappy. It could be to do with family or friends or school. No problem is too big or small for The Worry Tree. You can tell it anything you want and as much as you need to.

You tell the tree your worries. It feels like a great weight is lifting off you. You start to feel better straight away. You feel light and free and your mind becomes very clear. Your body feels relaxed and you feel very peaceful. It is a wonderful feeling to let your worries go. You thank the tree for taking your worries away.

Spend as long as you like relaxing peacefully under the Worry Tree and remember to come back anytime you need to...

I let my worries go
and feel
calm and free

Rainbow Thoughts

- *Worrying takes up time and energy. So let your worries go and feel the increase in your energy levels.*

- *Sometimes writing your worries down is a good way to let them go and free your mind.*

- *When you let go of your worries you free up your mind to be more focused and to concentrate on other things.*

- *Letting go can sometimes be hard-but the more you practice the better you get.*

Forest of Echoes

Imagine that you are standing in a forest. You are surrounded by huge trees and lots of forest scrub. It is a warm sunny day and the sky is clear and blue. You can see the sunlight peeking through the leaves and making patterns on the forest floor. What else can you see?

You take a deep breath in and let the fresh clean smell of the forest fill your lungs. You listen to the sounds around you. Perhaps you can hear a bird chirping in the distance? It is very peaceful and relaxing in the forest. You feel very safe and secure.

As you walk along, enjoying the sights and sounds, a friendly little bird lands on your shoulder. The bird tells you that this is the forest of echoes. Anything that you say will be repeated back, over and over like an echo. The only rule is that is has to be something positive about yourself.

You like this idea and decide you will give it a try. You try something simple to start with *I am brave.* You say it out loud in the forest and wait. You hear *I am brave, I am brave, I am brave, I am brave, I am brave* as it echoes back through the forest.

The echo sounds amazing. It feels like the words vibrate right through you. It sounds like your voice only much deeper. It feels like all the trees in the forest have joined in with you and have sent the words back your way.

Now think of another positive affirmation or say something positive about yourself. When you are ready, say it aloud in the forest. Now listen carefully for the echo.

You feel really happy. The words make you feel energised and full of confidence. It is like the echo has helped to clear away any doubts or negative feelings that you had. You start to believe the words you are saying.

Try it again and remember it will only echo if you are using positive words or affirmations.

Spend as long as you like exploring the Forest of Echoes and remember you can come back and visit anytime you wish...

I believe in myself
and I feel my
confidence growing

Rainbow Thoughts

- *Using empowering words and affirmations can help make you feel better.*

- *We create what we think about. Make your thoughts, words and beliefs positive so that you create positive energy around you.*

- *Positive self talk helps us to feel more confident.*

- *Repeating words or affirmations helps to reinforce them. Repeat them as often as you can during the day.*

GREEN

Green is a balancing colour.
Green is the colour of
love and forgiveness.
Green helps us to
love ourselves
and others.

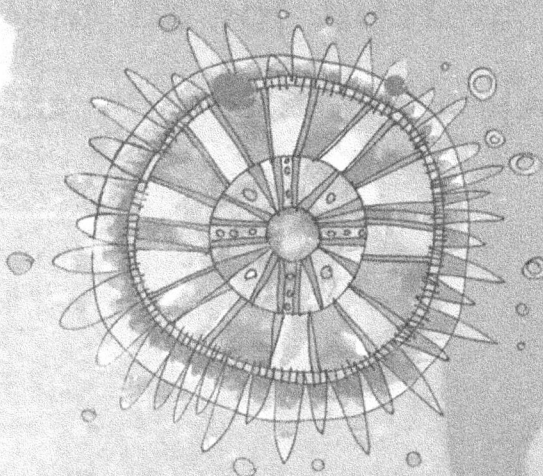

Green Affirmations

I am forgiving

I am thoughtful

I love myself

I am loving

I make friends easily

I am kind

I am caring

I am loved

I am balanced

I am grateful for all things

I enjoy the colour green

Green

Imagine that you are sitting on a comfortable chair in the centre of a room. This room is a special room. When you say a colour, the whole room turns that colour. Today your colour is green. You say the word *green* and watch as the room now turns completely green. First the walls turn green, then the ceiling, the floor, even the chair you are sitting on. It is as if the whole room is bathed in green light. Take a moment to look around the room. What else do you see? Put your hand into the green light. What does the colour green feel like?

You take a deep breath in through your nose, and then let it go out through your mouth. You count in two, three, and four and out two, three, and four. As you breathe in, imagine that the colour green is coming up from the floor of the room through the bottom of your feet. Every time you take a breath in, the colour spreads further up through your body. It is as if you are breathing in the colour green. What does the colour green smell like?

The colour spreads from the tips of your toes, up your legs, over your hips and stomach, up your chest, over your arms and fingers, up through your neck and shoulders, over your face until it reaches the top of your head and you are completely green. How does the colour green make you feel? What thoughts or ideas come to you when you are the colour green?

Spend as long as you like enjoying the colour green...

I enjoy
the colour
green

Rainbow Thoughts

- *Colour can be used to heal our body.*

- *Green is a balancing colour and good to use when you are feeling stressed.*

- *Green is said to create harmony and is the colour of nature.*

- *The colour green is soothing to the mind and body.*

- *Green is the colour of love and forgiveness.*

The Healing Pond

Imagine that you are standing at the edge of a big pond. The pond is in a small clearing in the bush and is completely surrounded by big trees and lots of greenery. What else can you see around your pond? It is very quiet and peaceful at the pond and although you are far away from anyone else, you feel very safe and secure. You listen carefully. It is so still, you can just hear some crickets and birds in the distance. What else do you hear? You take a deep breath in and smell the air. It smells so clean and fresh.

You now turn your attention to the pond. The water is so still and clear that you can see the bottom of the pond. You can see the sand and small pebbles scattered along the bottom. Can you see anything else?

You take off your shoes and slowly put your toes into the water. The water is cool and refreshing and you notice that your toes are beginning to tingle. You take your foot out and the tingling stops. You put your foot in again and the tingling returns. Just as you are wondering what is making you tingle, a little cricket lands on you. The cricket tells you not to be afraid and that the pond is a special healing pond. It is where all the animals and insects come to drink and bathe when they are not feeling well or are feeling sad. The cricket tells you that you are more than welcome to enjoy the pond and its healing waters.

You thank the cricket and decide to take a swim in the pond. You walk forward into the pond. As each part of your body enters the water, you feel a soft tingling which makes you feel very relaxed. You scoop up some water in your hand and take a sip. You feel the tingle inside of you as it spreads to the top of your head and tips of your toes. It is as if all the cells in your body are being cleaned and revitalized by the magical water in the pond. You dive underwater and let the water completely cover you. What does it feel like? Can you feel the cool water on your skin?

You come to the surface and feel so refreshed. You lie on your back, floating in the pond. You look up at the sky and relax. All the aches and pains have gone from your body. All your worries and fears have drifted away, and any negative thoughts are gone. You feel so peaceful.

Spend as long as you like enjoying the pond's healing powers. You can come back any time you need to, especially if you are feeling unwell or out of sorts...

I am balanced

Rainbow Thoughts

- *If you are feeling out of sorts, you can use your mind to help change the way you are feeling.*

- *Try letting go of negative thoughts and thinking positive ones and you will feel much better.*

- *Our imagination is a powerful tool and we can use it to help us feel better.*

- *Water has a wonderful calming effect. If you are not feeling well or are feeling agitated or angry, have a shower or bath or spend time near the ocean, a lake, a pond or a river.*

Make a Friend

Imagine that you are standing in a supermarket. There are lots of shelves full of products and colourful stands with big display signs. Can you see the cash registers and brightly coloured shopping trolleys? Take a good look all around. What else do you see? You realise that this is no ordinary supermarket. This supermarket has some very different ingredients on the shelves. You look closer at the sign which says *Make a Friend*. You are going to buy the ingredients that you think will make a good friend.

Before you start buying, it might be a good idea to have a good look around first. You start to walk around the supermarket. There are aisles full of products. There are jars, packets, boxes and cans. They are all different colours, shapes and sizes just like friends. Take a look at the labels on the shelves. There are so many things to pick from.

There are jars labelled with such words as: *happy, forgiving, patient.* There are packets of *kindness, caring, happy, honesty.* There are cans of *laughter* and boxes of *fun* and so much more. What else can you see?

Spend some time thinking about your closest friends and what you like about them. What makes a good friend?

Now think about how many ingredients you are made of? Do you think you are a good friend? Is there any ingredient you would like a little more of? Take a few moments to think about it. Think about why you are a good friend.

When you are ready, get a shopping trolley and start your shopping. There are lots of other people in the store. They smile at you as you walk past. You are having fun in this shop. You might even make some new friends while you are here.

Spend as long as you like shopping in the supermarket. You can come back and visit any time you wish...

I enjoy making
new friends

Rainbow Thoughts

- *Friends come in all different shapes and sizes.*
  What they look like is not important.
  It is what is inside them that is important.

- *Different people have different qualities which make them unique.*
  It would be boring if everyone was the same.

- *Sometimes our friends are the complete opposite from us and that makes for a balanced friendship.*

Hidden Cottage

Imagine that you are standing in the middle of a forest. It is a fresh spring day and you can feel a gentle breeze blowing. Sunlight streams gently through the leaves of the trees and you can see little patches of sunshine on the forest floor. You look all around and see that big tall trees surround you. All you can see in the distance is lush green forest. It is very peaceful in the forest and you feel very calm and safe. You listen carefully and see what sounds you can hear. Can you hear all the different birds? Can you hear the sounds of the leaves rustling in the breeze? Perhaps you can hear a rabbit hopping through the scrub? You can hear a strange sound in the distance so you decide to investigate.

You walk a little further through the forest towards the sound. The sound gets louder and louder. It sounds like someone is crying? You follow the sound until you see what looks like a cottage in the distance. As you get closer you see that is it a pretty white cottage sitting in a small clearing. You can see a washing line and vegetables growing. You can also see someone sitting on the veranda of the cottage crying. It is hard to see who it is so you walk even closer so you can see who or what is sitting and crying.

You find a big, strange looking, very hairy creature. At first you are a little afraid and are not sure what to do. It looks like the creature has hurt its foot. A little blue bird lands on your shoulder and tells you that the creature is very gentle and helps to care for all the animals and birds in the forest. The bird tells you that the creature has a big thorn in its foot and none of them have been able to remove it. You decide to go and help the creature. You feel quite safe now that you have the little bird with you and that she has told you that the creature is very gentle. You ask the creature if it is okay to take out the thorn and the creature nods his head. You quickly remove the thorn and help wrap the creature's foot with a bandage. The creature stops crying and thanks you for your kindness. His foot feels so much better now. He tells you that nobody had come to help him as they were afraid of him because he looks so big and hairy. You spend time talking to your new friend.

You now find that you have lost your way back, and are not sure how to get home. Your new friend tells you not to worry, that he knows the forest very well and that he will take you back; - after all you have been very kind to him. You say thank you and decide to stay a little longer exploring all the sights and sounds of the forest with your new friend.

Spend as long as you like enjoying the forest and when you are ready your new friend will show you the way back...

I treat everyone
with love
and kindness

Rainbow Thoughts

- *What you give, you will receive back. If you want to be treated kindly then be kind to others.*

- *Never judge someone on looks alone. It is what is on the inside that counts.*

- *Try to practice an act of kindness everyday and see how good you feel.*

- *Discuss the meaning of "Don't judge a book by its cover".*

Heart Flower

Imagine that you are standing in a field full of flowers. There are so many different flowers of all shapes and colours. There are white flowers, pink flowers, red flowers and blue flowers. What other colours can you see? It is a fine sunny day and you are enjoying the sunlight as it gently warms your skin. You take a deep breath in and smell the fresh air and the scent of the flowers. What flowers can you smell?

You walk through the field until you come across a giant pink flower bud. Perhaps it is a rose bud or a lotus flower. You sit down quietly and look at the giant bud. Can you see all the petals gently wrapped around each other waiting to unfold? What else can you see? You gently touch your flower. It is soft and velvety. What else can you feel?

Now imagine that your heart is like this giant flower bud, with lots of petals waiting to unfold. You start to think about all the things you have in your life that you are grateful for. It may be your family, your pet, your friends or the house you live in. You may be grateful for the fresh air you breathe or for someone helping you. You may be grateful to yourself for having a healthy body and a wonderful mind that you can think with and make choices with, there are so many possibilities. Think of all the things you are grateful for and say thank-you.

You notice that each time you are grateful; the petals of your flower heart start to open out. If any petals will not open, take a deep breath in and keep thinking of more positive things about yourself and your life and say thank-you. The more grateful you are, the more and more petals open until your flower is in full bloom. You feel amazing when your flower is in full bloom. You feel happy and content. You feel light and free. How else do you feel?

Spend time relaxing in the field of flowers, thinking about all the wonderful things in your life and come back anytime you need...

I am grateful
for all I have
in my life

Rainbow Thoughts

- *Sometimes people focus so much on what they haven't got that they forget to appreciate all the wonderful things that they do have.*

- *There are so many things to be grateful for and writing them in a gratitude journal is a great way to remember.*

- *Try to think of something you are grateful for every night before you go to sleep. It is a great habit to get into.*

- *There is a saying "taking things for granted". Thinking about what you have to be grateful for helps you to focus on even the smallest of things such as water to drink and a bed to sleep in.*

- *Think about the things that you have taken for granted in your life and learn to appreciate them.*

BLUE

Blue is a calming colour.
Blue is the colour of
communication
and honesty.
Blue helps us to
express ourselves.

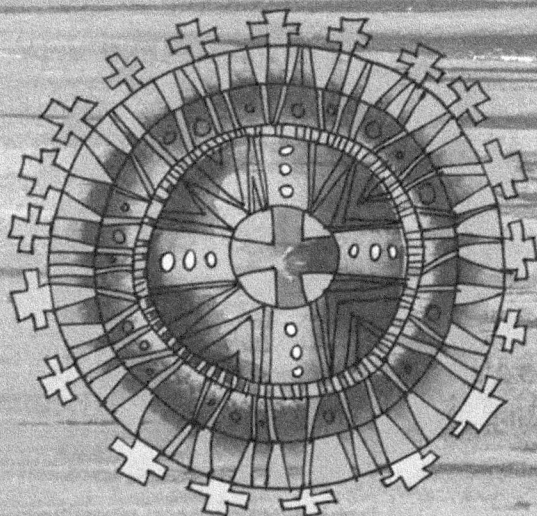

BLUE AFFIRMATIONS

I can express myself

I have choices

I am honest

I enjoy new experiences

I always speak from my heart

I listen

I am truthful

I am reliable

I trust my feelings and
listen to my heart

I enjoy the colour blue

Blue

Imagine that you are sitting on a comfortable chair in the centre of a room. This room is a special room. When you say a colour, the whole room turns that colour. Today your colour is blue. You say the word *blue* and watch as the room now turns completely blue. First the walls turn blue, then the ceiling, the floor, even the chair you are sitting on. It is as if the whole room is bathed in blue light. Take a moment to look around the room. What else do you see? Put your hand in the light. What does the colour blue feel like?

You take a deep breath in through your nose, and then let it go out through your mouth. You count in two, three, and four and out two, three, and four. As you breathe in imagine that the colour blue is coming up from the floor of the room through the bottom of your feet. Every time you take a breath in the colour spreads further up through your body. It is as if you are breathing in the colour blue. What does the colour blue smell like?

The colour spreads from the tips of your toes, up your legs, over your hips and stomach, up your chest, over your arms and fingers, up through your neck and shoulders, over your face until it reaches the top of your head and you are completely blue. How does the colour blue make you feel? What thoughts or ideas come to you when you are the colour blue?

Spend as long as you like enjoying the colour blue...

I enjoy

the colour

blue

Rainbow Thoughts

- *Colours can have an impact on our sense of well being.*

- *Blue is a calming colour. It is the colour of peace and tranquillity.*

- *Pale blue (along with pale green) is often used in hospitals and places of healing.*

- *Blue is a good colour for communication and listening.*

Whale Song

Imagine that you are sitting in a boat in the middle of a beautiful bay in the ocean. You look around and can see nothing but the beautiful blue ocean surrounding you. Behind you, you can just make out the shoreline and houses in the bay, but they seem very far away. It is a beautiful warm sunny day. The skies are clear and blue and the ocean is calm. You take in a big breath of fresh sea air. It is so clean and refreshing.

Look around your boat. It is a special boat used for studying marine life. It is a big white boat. It has a special viewing deck at the back with a glass bottom so that you can see below. The boat has its name on the side. Can you see what it is called? What else can you see on your boat?

You sit quietly on the deck taking in some deep breaths of fresh sea air when you hear a sound to your right. You look in the direction of the sound and see a beautiful humpback whale. The sound you have heard is the whale blowing water out of its blowhole. You look in amazement as the whale gently moves through the water. It is so big and graceful. You look carefully and see that there are several more whales near the boat. You can also see the water spurting out into the air from their blowholes. They are very curious mammals and have come to have a look at you and your boat. You feel very safe on your boat and you know that the whales are very gentle. Two big whales swimming together come right up to the boat. As they come close to the boat they turn on the backs and glide under the glass deck at the end of the boat. Can you see their big white bellies? What else can you see?

Another whale comes right up to the viewing deck. It is so close you can almost touch it. The whale pops its head out of the water and looks at you. It is as if the whale has come to say hello. The whale almost looks like it is smiling at you. These whales are very playful and they seem to sense that you are a friend. All of a sudden, with a big powerful arch, it dives away splashing its tail flukes onto the water. Seawater sprays all over you and onto the deck. It makes you laugh and it also makes you very wet. Can you feel the salty water on your skin? Can you see the whale flap its fin along the water? It looks like it is waving to you. What else can you see the whales doing?

You watch as the whales continue to play around the boat. You see a mother and baby. The mother whale is gently guiding its calf through the ocean. The calf swims very close to its mother. The whales all seem to be moving together in the same direction. Where do you think they are heading?

Perhaps you have a special underwater listening device on your boat. See if you can find it and listen carefully? Are they making any sounds? Can you hear them calling to each other? What else do you hear?

Spend as long as you like relaxing on the deck of your boat and watching the whales as they play together in the bay...

I enjoy taking the time to notice and listen

Rainbow Thoughts

- *Everyone communicates and interacts differently.*
- *Animals have special ways of interacting and communicating with each other.*
- *Different species of whales use varying methods of clicks and whistles and regular sounds of changing frequency to communicate. Some sing as a method of communicating.*
- *Think about all the ways humans can communicate.*
- *Sometimes when we sit back and observe quietly, we see and hear so much more.*
- *Being a really good listener is important.*

Waterfall

Imagine that you are standing in a beautiful rainforest at the base of a waterfall. You see the waterfall plunging over a rocky outcrop above and watch as it cascades down over rocks and into a giant pool. Can you hear the sound of the water as it rushes over the rocks and plunges into the pool? Can you see it swirling and the white froth it makes? You look closely at the giant pool. The water calms as it enters the pool and you notice it is a beautiful blue colour. You watch as the water moves from the pool across more rocks into a stream below. The water is shallow at the edges and you feel very safe.

You move closer to the waterfall until you feel the water spray as it lands on your skin. It feels very refreshing and soon your whole face is moist from the spray. You move closer again until you are standing under the waterfall. You feel the power of the water as it washes over your head and shoulders. You watch as the water gently dances over your body. You put your hands underneath and watch as the water bounces off them making different patterns in the pool below.

Imagine that the power from the waterfall is flowing though your whole body. It is so cool and refreshing and you feel the power spread from your head, down your neck and shoulders, to your arms, stomach, your legs and down to your feet and toes. As the water washes over you, you feel like all your worries are washing away.

Now think about any feelings you have that you don't like or that feel stuck inside you. Imagine the water clearing any blockages and moving them out of the body. Feel the water washing them away until you feel re-energised and clear. You continue this exercise until you feel a tingle in your throat. This tingle tells you that you are clear and free of any stuck feelings. How do you feel?

Spend as much time as you want enjoying the waterfall and swimming in the pool. You may return any time that you need to be re-energised and to clear your mind and body...

I am clear and free

to express my

feelings

Rainbow Thoughts

- *Try this visualisation in the shower. Imagine the water from the shower is the waterfall washing over you.*

- *Sometimes we have trouble expressing our feelings and they seem to be stuck inside us. If you visualise removing the blocks it can help you to express yourself better.*

- *If you have trouble expressing your feelings, try practising by talking in the mirror to yourself or saying them out loud in the form of an affirmation.*

- *Try saying this powerful affirmation: "It is safe for me to express how I feel."*

Underwater Cave

Imagine that you are standing on a beautiful beach. The sand is white and clean and it feels so soft beneath your toes. It is a warm sunny day and the sky is clear and blue. You can hear the sound of the waves as they gently break against the shore. What else can you hear? You take a look around you and notice that at one end of the beach there is a large rock formation just off the shore. You walk towards the rocks and as you get closer you can see that there is a small reef surrounding them. You walk out onto the reef. The water feels cool and refreshing. You notice that where the reef surrounds the rocks, there is a big pool of water. It almost looks like a swimming pool. It is an amazing blue colour and looks so inviting that you feel like going for a swim.

You look down into the water and see something coming towards you. It is a beautiful grey dolphin. The dolphin is a friendly dolphin and he tells you that his name is Nero. Nero invites you to come in for a swim with him and to visit the underwater cave. Nero tells you that you will be very safe and that you only have to hold your breath for a short time. You climb onto Nero's back and hold on to his fin. Nero feels slippery and wet. What else can you feel? You hold your breath and away you go.

Nero dives underwater and heads for the cave. It is an amazing feeling. The water rushes over you and you leave a trail of bubbles behind. You are having so much fun. You can see schools of fish dashing and darting around as you come towards them. What else do you see? Do you see the sea horses hiding in the seaweed?

You look ahead and see that you are heading towards the rocks. You can see that there is an opening in the rocks. Nero dives a little deeper to reach the opening and in you go. You keep holding on and before you know it you have surfaced. You take a big breath and look around you. You are in the underwater cave. The cave is huge. You realise that is must be in the centre of all the rocks you can see from the shore. You climb off Nero and onto the rocks. You thank Nero for bringing you here. The cave has the most amazing shiny stones and shells set into its walls. They are all different shapes and colours and textures. What else can you see?

It is nice and cool in your cave. Small streams of sunlight are peeking through the cracks in the rocks, bathing the cave in a warm, soft light. You see something in the corner. It is a special bed made out of seaweed. You decide to investigate.

You walk over and touch the bed. The seaweed feels very silky and smooth. You decide to lie down on the bed and see what it is like. It is so soft and comfortable that you sink right into the bed. Your mind feels so clear. Anything that is troubling you gently drifts away. It is so quiet and peaceful in the cave. You listen carefully and all that you can hear is the sound of your own breathing.

You feel very relaxed and very calm. You take a few more deep breaths and enjoy the feeling of being quiet. When you are quiet great ideas can pop into your head, or sometimes an answer to a problem may come to you. Take some more deep breaths and see what ideas come to you or think of a question and see what answers you get.

Spend as long as you like exploring your quiet cave. When you are ready Nero will take you back to the beach. You can come back any time you want to feel peaceful and quiet...

When I am quiet, I can hear the answers to my questions more easily

Rainbow Thoughts

- *It is ok to take time out on your own in a special place.*
- *Sometimes when we stop and are quiet, solutions come to us more easily.*
- *We may not have an underwater cave in real life but we can always visit the one in our mind.*
- *When we are calm and relaxed our mind has a chance to clear and we feel much better.*

Dragon Egg

Imagine that you are walking along a beach. It is a beautiful sunny day and you can feel the fresh sea air on your face. You take a deep breath in and let the clean salty air fill you lungs. You listen carefully and hear gulls overhead and small waves gently lapping at the shore. You enjoy the feeling of the sand as it gently massages your feet. The beach is surrounded by rocky cliffs. Can you see the small caves in the face of the cliffs? What else do you see?

You walk along the beach and look at all the things that are washed up on the shore. There are shells and rocks. Can you see all the different coloured seaweed? What else do you see? You keep looking along the beach and something ahead of you catches your eye. It is a blue shiny object. You get closer and pick it up. You realise it is a giant egg. It is unlike anything you have seen before. It is all different shades of blue in colour and glitters in the sunlight.

You hear a voice in your head say, Please *take me and put me some place warm*. You wonder who has spoken and you hear it again: *Please take me and put me some place warm.* You pick the egg up and wrap it in a towel. You take it to a small cave you have seen about half way up the cliff where the egg will be safe. The cave is warm and comfortable and very quiet. You will come back each day to visit and enjoy sitting in the peaceful cave and listening to the sound of the waves.

One day when you arrive you realise that the egg has hatched and sitting next to the empty shell is a baby dragon. It is very glad to see you and jumps into your arms and licks you all over your face. The little dragon wants to be your friend. You stroke the dragon from head to tail. The dragon's skin feels cool and smooth. He is different shades of blue and his scales glitter and sparkle. What else can you feel?

You spend time playing with your new friend and soon learn he can understand you. You have a special way of communicating: One snort means yes and two snorts means no. What tricks can you teach your dragon?

Your dragon is doubling in size every day and by the end of the week he is taller than you and ready to fly. After another week he is fully grown. Your dragon wants to take you flying. You hop on his back and hold on with a special harness and off you go. You feel very safe and secure on the back of your dragon. You feel the wind rushing over your face as your dragon ducks and dives. Your dragon seems to know where you want to go. You feel yourself laughing and feeling light and free. As you ride through the air all your worries seem to disappear. Your dragon is happy too. What do you see as you fly with your dragon?

You hear a voice talking to you in your mind. You listen carefully and realise that your dragon can read your thoughts and you can read his. Your dragon is talking to you. You seem to be able to communicate to each other by talking in your mind. Your dragon is very wise and can help you if you have anything that is worrying you. Try sending your dragon some messages and then spend a few moments taking some deep breaths and see if your dragon has any messages for you. You find it very easy to talk to your dragon and tell it how you are feeling.

Spend as long as you like playing with your dragon and enjoying this new way of communicating. You can come back any time you wish...

I enjoy new experiences

Rainbow Thoughts

- *New friends come in different shapes and sizes just like the big dragon.*
- *It is exciting to try new things, don't be afraid of change.*
  Trying new things can lead to new adventures.
- *Learning new things can help you to grow as a person.*
- *If you are kind and considerate to others then they are more likely to be kind and considerate back to you.*
- *You can always find a way to communicate with someone even if they don't speak the same language as you.*

INDIGO

Indigo is an intuitive colour.
Indigo is the colour of
wisdom
and imagination.
Indigo helps us to see
in meditation.

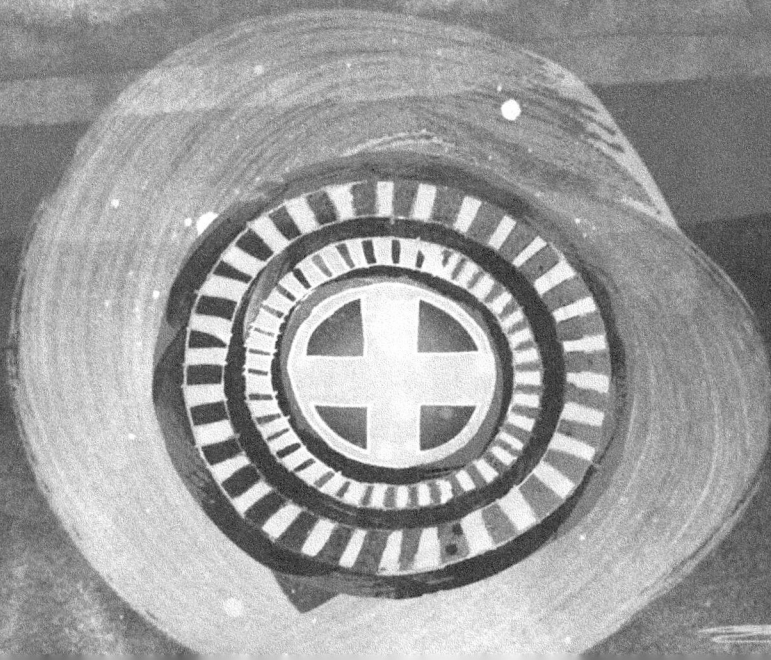

INDIGO AFFIRMATIONS

I trust my feelings

I am peaceful

I am full of wisdom

I learn from my mistakes

I have a great imagination

I use my imagination
to achieve great things

I see the good in others

I enjoy being quiet

I make good decisions

I enjoy the colour Indigo

Indigo

Imagine that you are sitting on a comfortable chair in the centre of a room. This room is a special room, when you say a colour, the whole room turns that colour. Today your colour is Indigo. You say the word *Indigo* and watch as the room now turns a deep blue almost dark purple colour called Indigo. First the walls turn Indigo, then the ceiling, the floor, even the chair you are sitting on. It is as if the whole room is bathed in Indigo light. Take a moment to look around the room. What else do you see? Put your hand into the Indigo light. What does the colour Indigo feel like?

You take a deep breath in through your nose, and then let it go out through your mouth. You count in two, three, and four and out two, three, and four. As you breathe in imagine that the colour Indigo is coming up from the floor of the room through the bottom of your feet. Every time you take a breath in the colour spreads further up through your body. It is as if you are breathing in the colour Indigo. What does the colour Indigo smell like?

The colour spreads from the tips of your toes, up your legs, over your hips and stomach, up your chest, over your arms and fingers, up through your neck and shoulders, over your face until it reaches the top of your head and you are completely indigo.

How does the colour Indigo make you feel? What thoughts or ideas come to you when you are the colour Indigo?

Spend as long as you like enjoying the colour Indigo...

I enjoy
the colour
Indigo

Rainbow Thoughts

- *Each colour has its own wavelength and its own energy.*

- *Indigo is a very good colour to open up our intuition and to tap into our imagination.*

- *Indigo is a good colour to helps us get to sleep. It has a calming sedative affect.*

Peaceful Cloud

Imagine that you are sitting on top of a cloud watching the sun set. Your cloud is white and fluffy and feels so soft to touch. Even though you are high above the ground, you feel very safe and secure sitting on your cloud. It is a warm day and you watch as sun slowly disappears and the sky changes colour. It goes from pale blue to shades of orange, pink and violet. You have a fantastic view from your cloud and you feel very relaxed watching the beautiful warm colours change the colour of the sky. You watch the last bit of sun slip below the horizon and decide to lie down on your cloud.

You lie back and feel the soft cloud all around you. It is like lying on a bed of giant cotton wool. It is so comfortable. You take a few deep breaths. You breathe in two, three, and four and out two, three, and four. You feel your body sink further into the cloud. It is so quiet and peaceful on your cloud. You listen carefully and can hear nothing but the sound of your own breathing. You look above you and watch as the sky turns to night. The violet sky becomes blue again. You watch as the blue gets darker and darker until it becomes a beautiful Indigo colour. Small stars start to twinkle and sparkle in the night sky. How many can you count? Can you see any shapes or patterns?

One small twinkling star catches your eye. It looks like it is moving. You watch as it starts to come closer and closer. You realise that it is coming towards you. The little star stops right above you. It sprinkles shiny stardust all over your body. It tickles and tingles as it lands gently on your body. You take a deep breath in and feel your legs relax and sink into the cloud. With your next breath your hips relax and sink into the cloud. Then your stomach, your arms and your chest relax and sink into the cloud. The little star then sprinkles some stardust on your forehead. The stardust makes your face feel very soft and relaxed. You feel very still and peaceful. Your eyes get heavier and heavier and you feel very sleepy. You hear the star tell you to dream magical dreams and have a wonderful rest.

Spend as long as you like relaxing and sleeping peacefully on your cloud...

I enjoy being quiet

Rainbow Thoughts

- *We can use our imagination to take us places at any time of the day.*

- *Try lying outside watching the stars at night and you will see how relaxing it is.*

- *It is good to calm our overactive minds by spending some quiet time every day.*

Inner Temple

Imagine that you are standing in a beautiful big park. It is a warm sunny day and the sky is clear and blue. There is a gentle breeze blowing. You look around the park and see lots of big green trees and soft green grass. There are benches for people to sit on and beautiful flower gardens to enjoy. Can you see the big playground with swings and climbing equipment? There is a big yellow slide that finishes in a big sandpit full of soft white sand and a blue see-saw. There are wooden tables and chairs to sit at and enjoy a picnic. What else can you see? You take a deep breath in and let the fresh air fill your lungs. You notice a path winding through the park and you decide to follow it. You step onto the path and walk past a beautiful rose garden. There are pink roses, yellow roses, red roses and white roses all in bloom. Can you smell their perfume in the air?

You keep walking on your path through all the beautiful trees until your path leads you to a gigantic pond, right in the centre of the park. In the middle of the pond there is an island with a white building on it. There is a wooden bridge leading across the pond to the building. Do you see it? You decide to walk across the bridge to investigate further. Once you have crossed the bridge you notice that it has disappeared. A little bird lands on your shoulder and tells you that this is your own special place, and only you can cross the bridge. When you are ready to leave it will reappear. You thank the little bird and walk towards the white building.

You open the door and step inside. It is so quiet and peaceful. There are soft white cushions on the floor and sheer white curtains covering the windows. It is like your own special temple. You sit on the cushions and take some deep breaths. It is so quiet that all you can hear is the sound of your own breath. You watch as the curtains gently move in and out. You notice that the curtains seem to move in and out with each breath you take. It is as if you are part of the temple. You take a moment to be mindful of your surroundings. What does your temple smell like? Perhaps it is your favourite smell? What do the cushions feel like beneath you?

You continue to take some deep breaths. You feel your body relax and all your muscles soften. You feel all your worries and thoughts gently drifting away. Your mind feels still and clear. Your whole body feels so calm and relaxed. It is a very peaceful feeling. You repeat to yourself *I am calm, I am calm, I am calm.*

While you are calm and relaxed in your temple you will be able to hear your inner wisdom. Think of a question you need to ask or a problem you need a solution to and ask. See what answer comes to mind. Now concentrate on how you feel with this answer and trust the feelings you are receiving, this is your inner wisdom talking. You will feel deep down inside if this is the correct response for you. Ask as many questions as you need to.

Spend as long as you like in your special temple enjoying the quiet, peaceful feeling and remember that you can come back here any time you wish...

I enjoy spending quiet time
on my own

Rainbow Thoughts

- *Sometimes when things are bothering you it is good to visit your own quiet space.*

- *Being quiet and spending time alone each day doesn't mean you are lonely - you are getting to know yourself better.*

- *You can visit your quiet temple whenever you wish. Just tap into your imagination or listen to your inner wisdom.*

- *After spending quiet time and clearing your thoughts you will find that it is easier to explore your imagination and listen to your inner wisdom.*

- *Learn to trust your "gut feelings" or inner wisdom.*

- *Do what you think is the right thing, not what others want you to do.*

Picture Frame

Imagine that you are standing in the entrance of a beautiful art gallery. The gallery is so big and spacious. It has magnificent high ceilings, and all the walls and ceilings are painted white. The gallery has polished wooden floors and there are beautiful lights throughout the ceiling. They look like stars twinkling in the night sky. You look all around you and see that the art gallery is full of wonderful paintings. They are all hanging on the crisp white walls. There are so many different paintings with such amazing colours. You see a sign saying, *Please Enjoy Visiting the most Amazing Places in the World,* and you decide to enter.

You walk around the gallery looking at the paintings. The first one you see is a painting of a beautiful cottage and its garden. The cottage is blue and has a white picket fence. There are so many flowers and birds and butterflies. What else do you see? If you look closely at the picture you can see there is a table in the garden and on the table is a plate of scones with jam and cream. There is also a little bridge that passes over a huge pond full of lilies. Can you see the frogs sitting on them?

The next picture is of a field of sunflowers. It is so bright and happy looking. There are hundreds of yellow sunflowers with their petals wide open facing the sun. You feel warm just looking at the picture. In the background you can see a little farmhouse with a green tractor parked at the side. The closer you look at the paintings, the more details you can see.

You keep walking around the gallery. There are paintings of deserts and beautiful tropical islands. There are jungles, rainforests and ancient temples. There are paintings of the beach and of beautiful castles. There are bush scenes and snow scenes. There are mountains, lakes and rivers. What other paintings can you see? What amazing colours do they have?

You come to the last picture in the gallery and find that it is blank. Next to it is a set of paints and a brush. There is also a sign saying, *It's your turn to paint an amazing place.* Think about your magical place and then say *I am Creative.*

You think about an amazing place you have been or maybe it is somewhere that you would like to visit. You say to yourself *I am Creative.* As you say the words something magical happens. The paint brush starts painting all on its own. It is painting from the ideas you are thinking about. It is as if your imagination is painting the picture for you. The more ideas you have, the faster the brush moves. So many wonderful ideas come to you and you watch as your painting takes shape.

Your picture is finally finished and you stand back and take a look. What a beautiful picture and what a clever, inventive person you are. You reach forward to touch your painting, and as you do something amazing happens. It is as if you can not only see the scene, but you can touch it, taste it and smell it. You look all around you and realise that you are actually standing in the scene you have painted. Your painting has come to life. You can now explore your painting and all the wonderful things you have created.

When you are ready just say the word *back* and you will return to the art gallery. You can also explore any of the other paintings in the gallery. Just gently touch it and it will come to life.

Spend as long as you like in the art gallery enjoying all the amazing places you can visit...

I have a wonderful imagination

Rainbow Thoughts

- *Our imagination is limitless and the more we use it the better we get at it.*
- *Using our imagination helps us to become creative thinkers and increases our problem solving skills.*
- *Your imagination can help turn your thoughts into reality.*
- *Discuss this quote from Albert Einstein:*
  "Imagination is everything. It is the preview of life's coming attractions".

The Magic Factory

Imagine that you are standing in the middle of a huge factory. This is no ordinary factory. It is the magic factory where they make everything that is magical. The factory is so big and colourful. It has a red roof, yellow walls and bright green stairs. All the floors are purple and all the doors are orange. You can see big pots bubbling away and jars of lotions and potions on the shelves. What else can you see? Can you see the little elves tending to the pots? Can you see the fairies labelling the jars? They are all wearing little aprons and hats made out of a shiny violet material. They wave to you and tell you that the factory is yours to explore and to have a good time.

You start to look around the factory. All the rooms have big glass windows so that you can see inside. You watch carefully as you go to each room, there are so many new things to learn. There is a special room in the factory where they make wands and broomsticks, and a room where they keep all the books with the spells and potions in them. What other rooms can you see? Can you see the candy room where the Gnomes are busy making all kinds of different lollies and chocolates. You take a deep breath in. What does it smell like? Each candy does something magical. Some candies help you to fly and other candies turn you invisible. Pick one up and take a bite. What does it taste like? What magical thing happens to you?

The gnomes invite you to come and learn how to make some of the potions that they sell in the magic shop. You watch and listen carefully. They teach you how to make a magic potion that makes you sing like an opera star. You drink a bit and test your voice. How do you sound?

You see a big ladder and decide to investigate. You climb up the ladder to the shelves where all the jars of lotions and potions are kept. You see beautiful glass jars full of all different colours. You pick one jar up and read the label. It says *Rainbow.* You take the lid off to look inside and to your amazement a beautiful big rainbow comes out and lights up the whole room. It seems to shimmer and sparkle and then dance across the factory floor. What else can you see on the shelf? You pick up the jar with *Snow* written on it. You open the lid and there is a big whirl of white that goes right up to the top of the factory. It starts to snow inside and you watch as the snowflakes softly land, covering the factory in a soft white coating. What other jars can you see on the shelves? Pick another one to open and watch what happens.

Spend as long as you like having fun in the Magic Factory. You can come back and visit any time you wish...

My imagination is limitless

Rainbow Thoughts

- *Using your imagination and being creative helps you to see things in new ways.*

- *One of our most powerful gifts is our imagination.*

- *Develop your imagination. Visualise for yourself.*
  Don't rely on television or electronics to visualise for you.

VIOLET

Violet is a peaceful colour.
Violet is the colour of
spirituality
and connection.
Violet helps us to feel
a part of something great.

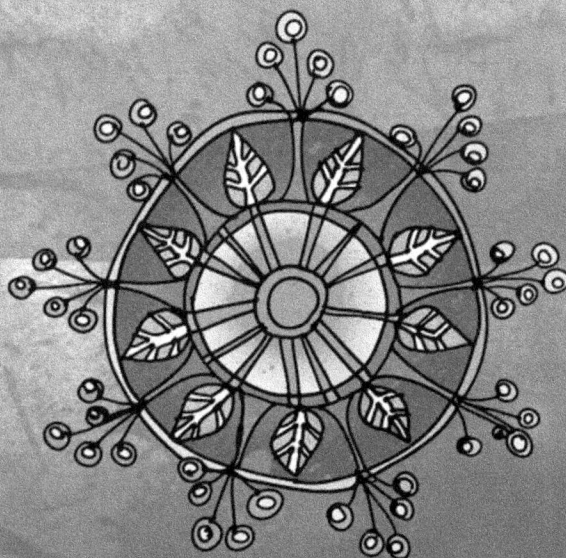

Violet Affirmations

I am perfect

I am beautiful

I am unique

I am free

I believe in me

My dreams come true

I accept myself

I create my happiness

I am perfect the way that I am

I enjoy the colour violet

Violet

Imagine that you are sitting on a comfortable chair in the centre of a room. This room is a special room, when you say a colour, the whole room turns that colour. Today your colour is Violet. You say the word *violet* and watch as the room now turns to violet. First the walls turn violet, then the ceiling, the floor, even the chair you are sitting on. It is as if the whole room is bathed in violet light. Take a moment to look around the room. What else do you see? Put your hand into the violet light. What does the colour violet feel like?

You take a deep breath in through your nose, and then let it go out through your mouth. You count in two, three, and four and out two, three, and four. As you breathe in imagine that the colour violet is coming up from the floor of the room through the bottom of your feet. Every time you take a breath in the colour spreads further up through your body. It is as if you are breathing in the colour violet. What does the colour violet smell like?

The colour spreads from the tips of your toes, up your legs, over your hips and stomach, up your chest, over your arms and fingers, up through your neck and shoulders, over your face until it reaches the top of your head and you are completely violet. How does the colour violet make you feel? What thoughts or ideas come to you when you are the colour violet?

Spend as long as you like enjoying the colour violet...

ɪ enjoy
the colour
violet

Rainbow Thoughts

- *Colour can affect our spiritual self.*

- *Violet has the highest energy and shortest wavelength of all the spectral colours.*

- *Violet is a good colour to help us feel connected and to be aware of what is going on around us.*

- *Violet is a very calming colour and is related to self-knowledge.*

Snow Sled

Imagine that you are standing on top of a huge mountain. It is covered in soft white snow. You take a deep breath in and feel the fresh cool air fill your lungs. You pick up some snow in your hand. What does if feel like? There is a light breeze blowing and you feel it as it passes, gently tickling your face. The clouds are so close that you can reach out and touch them. You take a good look all around you. The view from the mountain is breathtaking. Do you see the rooftops of the houses in the village below? They look like tiny little spots in the distance. Can you see the trees growing on the side of the mountain? Some of the trees have snow on the tips of their leaves. They look like they have been dipped in white. What else do you see? Are there any animals or birds on the mountain? Look very carefully you may see a long-eared rabbit hopping through the snow or a fox darting through the grass.

You see a snow sled in front of you. What colour is it? What is it made of? You hop into the snow sled and put your safety belt on. You see a pair of goggles and put these on too. They will protect your eyes from the wind and snow. You say these magic *words I am free, I am free, I am free* and you feel the sled start to move. You hold on tight to the steering wheel and off you go.

The sled starts to pick up speed but you feel very safe. You glide past trees and feel the wind whooshing on your face. Your hair is flying behind you in the wind. What else do you feel? Do you feel the snow flicking onto you? What can you see as you wind down the mountain?

You are having so much fun and enjoying every moment. You can feel that you have a big smile on your face. As the sled is weaving its way down the mountain you have not a care in the world. It is just you and your sled enjoying this beautiful winter day. It goes from left to right and back again, making a wonderful zigzag pattern in the snow.

When you get to the bottom, your sled slows down to a halt. You have arrived at the village you saw from the top of the mountain. You see that there is a special chair lift to take you and your sled back to the top of the mountain when you are ready or maybe you would like to go and explore the village and have a nice hot chocolate. It is up to you.

Spend as long as you like enjoying the mountain and playing in the snow...

I enjoy being free

Rainbow Thoughts

- *We learn a lot about ourselves when we try new and challenging things.*

- *Exercise is not only good for us but has a calming effect on our body. If you are ever feeling "off" try going for a walk or doing some form of exercise.*

- *When we feel free, we are more open to learning things and we understand ourselves better.*

- *Enjoy each moment as it happens. Don't worry about what is going to happen next or you will spend all your time thinking and none enjoying.*

Sinking Stone

Imagine that you are floating in a crystal clear pool of water. This pool is full of fresh spring water that comes down from the mountains. The pool is surrounded by beautiful trees and the sunlight peeks through the leaves and seemingly dances across the water's surface. The water feels cool and refreshing as it gently soothes your back. You feel very safe just relaxing in the pool of water. You look up at the sky and watch as wisps of clouds gently float by. Can you see any patterns in the clouds? You continue floating, enjoying the feeling of being weightless.

As you relax floating in the pond, imagine that your body starts to feel heavier. The heavy feeling starts in your stomach and chest, it slowly spreads to your arms and hands, your legs and feet, and finally to your neck and head. Even your mouth and eyes feel heavy. You feel yourself slowly and gently start to sink. You feel very safe and even though you are sinking you find you can still breathe.

You watch as the water slowly covers your body. You feel something solid underneath you and slowly come to a stop. The pool of water is not very deep and you are now comfortably resting on the bottom. It is so quiet and peaceful. You can still breathe easily and enjoy the complete silence. When you look up you can still see the sky through the water and rays of sunlight are making the water twinkle. The water is so clear and clean. What else do you see?

You continue to relax and feel all the tension and stress leave your body. All your thoughts and worries seem to vanish while you are gently resting on the bottom of the pool. You rest in complete silence, enjoying the peace and quiet. Your mind feels calm and clear. You feel free and your body feels light.

Spend as long as you like enjoying the beautiful mountain pool. When you are ready, gently float back to the surface. You can come back any time you wish...

I enjoy the feeling
of being free

Rainbow Thoughts

- *We do not get to relax in complete silence very often.*
  Try doing it for five minutes and see how it makes you feel.

- *Sometimes we need a complete break from all the noise and everything going on around us.*

- *Practising a few minutes of complete silence with some deep breaths is very good before you are doing a creative activity, learning something new or doing an exam or test. It helps to clear the mind so new ideas have space to develop and the knowledge that you have can easily be tapped in to.*

- *Quiet time allows your mind the time to sort through all your thoughts and feelings.*

Moon Bathing

Imagine that you are lying on a soft comfortable bed. It is night time and you are getting ready to go to sleep. You are wearing soft comfortable clothing and have your arms relaxed by your side with your palms facing upwards. You take some long deep breaths. You look up at the ceiling and notice that something is starting to form right in the centre above your bed. You watch as a beautiful glass dome appears. You can stars twinkling in the night sky.

You notice that the room is bathed in soft white moonlight. The moonlight is streaming through the dome and completely bathes you from the top of your head to the tips of your toes. The moonlight feels warm and is very calming. You feel very safe and your body starts to feel all soft and jelly-like. The moonlight continues to bathe you and you feel all your worries disappear. Your mind feels clear and free.

The moon tells you to look up into the sky and it will show you a picture of a very special person, someone who is perfect just the way they are. You look up at the moon and see your own face smiling back at you.

The moon whispers some messages to you and asks you to repeat what it says;

The moon tells you that you are unique.
You repeat *I am unique*
The moon tells you that you are one of a kind.
You repeat *I am one of a kind*
The moon tells you that you are safe and loved.
You repeat *I am safe and loved*
The moon tells you to believe in yourself.
You repeat *I believe in me*

Your mouth softens, your eyes become very heavy and sleepy. The moon whispers to you to believe in your dreams and they will come true.

You repeat *My dreams come true.*
You feel very happy and relaxed.

Spend as long as you like bathing in the moonlight and remember you can have a moonlight bath anytime you wish...

I am special and unique, there is no-one else like me

Rainbow Thoughts

- *You can have a moon bath whenever you are having trouble getting to sleep or you are not feeling good about yourself.*

- *If you believe in yourself you can be anything you want to be.*

- *Try repeating positive affirmations whenever you can.*

- *Enjoy being, feeling and thinking positively and you will attract like-minded friends and be happier.*

- *Learn to love yourself for who you are, don't try and change to suit others.*

Sleeping Lotus

Imagine you are sitting in the middle of a giant lotus flower. It has beautiful long white petals. The flower is very soft and comfortable. You feel warm and safe sitting inside it. It is so quiet and peaceful in the flower that you decide to lie on your back and have a rest. You close your eyes and take some deep breaths. You breathe in and out. The Lotus tells you that if you listen carefully it will help you to relax.

A soft white petal closes across your feet. The petal is so soft and the minute it touches your skin you feel a warm tingle in your feet and you hear the flower whisper: *Your feet are relaxed.* You feel your feet go soft and sink into the flower.

A second white petal closes across your legs. The warm tingle starts in your legs. You hear the flower whisper: *Your legs are relaxed.* You feel your legs go soft and sink into the flower.

A third white petal closes across your hips. The warm tingle moves across your hips and you hear the flower whisper: Your *hips are relaxed.* You feel your hips go soft and sink into the flower.

A fourth white petal closes across your stomach and you feel the warm tingle. The flower whispers: *Your stomach is relaxed.* You feel your stomach relax and sink towards the flower.

A fifth white petal closes across your chest. The warm tingle begins and the flower whispers: *Your chest is relaxed.* You feel your chest go soft and sink towards the flower.

A sixth white petal closes across your shoulders and arms and you feel the warm tingle. The flower whispers: *Your shoulders and arms are relaxed.* You feel your shoulders and arms go soft and sink into the flower.

The last petal closes across your forehead. Your head tingles with a nice warmth. The flower whispers: *Your mind is relaxed.* You feel your face relax and your mouth soften. Any worries or troubles seem to disappear. Your mind becomes clear and you feel very peaceful and relaxed. The petals feel like a light doona gently covering you.

You continue to take some deep breaths and enjoy the feeling of being warm, safe and still.

Spend as long as you like relaxing in the giant lotus and remember you can come back and visit anytime you need to relax and to enjoy being still...

I sleep peacefully
and dream magical dreams

Rainbow Thoughts

- *If we can find a calm space inside our mind, it does not matter what is going on around us, we can always visit it.*

- *Getting a good night's sleep is very important.*
  It allows our bodies to recharge for the next day.

- *If you are having trouble sleeping try saying some affirmations such as:*
  I sleep peacefully, I dream magic dreams, I am safe and protected,
  I feel peaceful and sleepy.

RAINBOW

Rainbows are a gift from nature.

The colours of the rainbow are very healing.

Rainbows bring joy to those who see them.

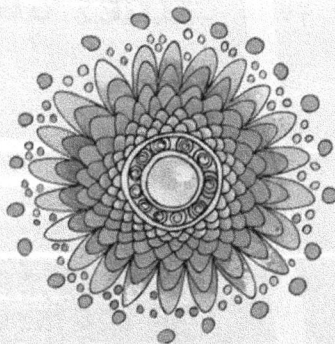

Rainbow Affirmations

I see magic everywhere

I am balanced

I always take time to relax

I create harmony in my life

I enjoy growing and changing

I learn something new every day

I am connected to all life on earth

I listen to my body

I love myself just how I am

I am full of energy

I honour my values and beliefs

The Affirmation Garden

Imagine that you are standing next to a beautiful sparkling pond. The water is so clear and still that it looks like a mirror. You look into the pond and see a very clear picture of yourself. How do you look? Do you look happy or sad?

The pond tells you that it is a magical pond and it is part of a wonderful garden. The pond whispers to you that you may take a walk in its garden. It tells you to follow the stepping stones on the ground and to repeat each message on your stepping stone aloud. You realise that you have found the magical affirmation garden.

As soon as you enter your garden you feel calm and relaxed. All the stress and tension leaves your body and you feel very, very safe. You look down on the ground and see the stepping stones. Each stepping stone has something different written on it. You repeat each message;

I am safe, I am healthy, I am strong, I am grateful.

You start to feel really good inside. You look around the garden and it seems to be bursting with red. You can see that all the flowers have opened. There are so many flowers all blooming in beautiful shades of red. There are red ladybirds and red beetles. There are little birds with red feathers, red apples and strawberries growing. What else can you see? What sounds can you hear? What can you smell?

You now walk to the next section of the garden. You repeat each message;

I am creative, I am happy, I am worthy, I enjoy having fun.

You feel really happy. Your garden starts to bloom with bright orange. There are pansies, carrots, mandarins and oranges growing everywhere. You see a beautiful orange butterfly flutter across the flowers and trees. What else can you see? What sounds can you hear?

You keep walking along your path and you come to the next set of stepping stones. You repeat each message;

I am valuable, I am confident, I think positive thoughts, I respect myself, I have potential.

You start to feel really confident inside. Your garden bursts into gold around you. Sunflowers bloom, there are daffodils, lemons, and you see a beautiful yellow bird sitting on a branch. What else can you see? What sounds can you hear?

You keep walking on your path and you come to the next set of stepping stones. You repeat each message;

I am forgiving, I am thoughtful, I love myself, I am loving, I make friends easily.

You start to feel really warm inside. Your garden bursts into pink and the green of the leaves seems brighter and brighter. Pink roses, pink petunias and carnations are all in bloom and you see little green frogs sitting on leaves smiling at you. What else can you see? What sounds can you hear?

You keep walking on your path and you come to the next set of stepping stones. You repeat each message;

I can express myself, I have choices, I am honest, I enjoy new experiences.

You feel a tingle in your throat. Your garden bursts into all the different shades of blue. Bluebells tinkle, blue butterflies appear all around you, little blue birds start to sing. What else can you see? What sounds can you hear?

You keep walking on your path and you come to the next set of stepping stones. You repeat each message;

I am peaceful, I am full of wisdom, I learn from my mistakes, I have a great imagination.

You feel amazing. Your garden bursts into the colours of indigo and dark purple. Deep dark blue flowers that look like the colour of the night fill the garden. Irises suddenly appear, pansies pop up everywhere. You can see the eggplants, mulberries, grapes and beetroots growing everywhere. What else can you see? What sounds can you hear?

You keep walking on your path and you come to the last set of stepping stones. You repeat each message;

I am perfect, I am beautiful, I am unique, I am free, I believe in me.

You feel radiant and full of joy. Your garden bursts into the colours of violet and white. Little violets and lilacs start to bloom, daisies appear, and there are roses and jasmine blooming everywhere. You can see little white butterflies dancing on the plump cauliflowers and so much more. What else can you see? What sounds can you hear?

You keep walking till you are back at the pond. What a wonderful time you have had enjoying all the magical rainbow colours of the garden. You look into the pond and see your reflection smiling back at yourself. How do you look? Do you see the big smile on your face? The pond whispers to you that it has a final message. It is a special message just for you? Look carefully into the pond and see if you can read it? What does it say?

Spend as long as you like relaxing in the Affirmation Garden. You can visit it whenever you wish...

I see magic everywhere

Rainbow Thoughts

- *Spending time in nature can make you feel better.*

- *Take the time to look at everything that is around you. There is magic everywhere. Enjoy the sights, sounds, smells and colours.*

- *When you are outside in nature, close your eyes and take some deep breaths. Listen to all the different sounds.*

- *Thoughts can be changed. You can change your mood and create your own happiness by using positive talk and thinking positive thoughts or doing something that you really enjoy.*

The Dragon's Cave

Imagine that you are standing in a clearing in the woods. You can see trees and shrubs. What else can you see? Can you see the big rocks? A sparkling waterfall runs over the rocks and into a small stream. You look closely and realise that at the centre of the rocks, just behind the waterfall is a large cave. You run your hand through the waterfall. It feels so cool and refreshing. You look into the waterfall and see something sparkling and decide to investigate.

You step through the waterfall and into the cave. The cave is covered in hundreds of beautiful crystals. They glitter and glow in all the colours of the rainbow. The crystals are red, orange, yellow, green, blue, indigo and violet, all in different shapes and sizes.

You look around and suddenly stop. There, in the middle of the cave, resting on a bed of crystals is a great dragon. The Dragon tells you not to be afraid; he is friendly and he has been waiting to meet you.

You slowly move forward and sit by the dragon. You pat him gently. His skin is like velvet and his scales glisten in the light. What else can you feel? You feel warm and safe as you sit by his side. The Dragon tells you about an ancient ceremony that only dragons know of that will make you feel fantastic.

The Dragon asks you to lie on his crystal bed. The Dragon tells you to relax and listen to the sound of your breathing. You breathe in through your nose and out through your mouth. You watch as the Dragon takes out a beautiful wooden box. As he opens the box a rainbow appears from inside. The Dragon shows you the source of the rainbow. Lying in the box are seven magnificent crystals, each one shining its beautiful coloured light.

The dragon places a magic red crystal at your feet. The light from the crystal shines brightly. The red crystal makes you feel strong and full of energy. You feel like your feet are growing roots into the ground. The red colour makes you feel safe and the dragon whispers to you: *You are Safe.* You repeat, *I am Safe.*

Next the dragon places an orange crystal just below your belly button. You feel the orange colour spread all over you. It makes you feel happy and full of good ideas. The dragon whispers to you: *You are happy.* You repeat, *I am happy.*

Next, the dragon places a yellow crystal onto your belly button; you feel a tingle spread throughout your body. The yellow crystal makes you feel strong and powerful. The dragon whispers a special message: *You are strong.* You repeat, *I am strong.*

Then the dragon does something amazing. He places a green crystal on your heart and very gently blows a ring of pink smoke across your body. It feels so good that your heart begins to feel warm and you can hear it beating gently. You think about all the people that love you. The dragon whispers a special message: *You are loved.* You repeat, *I am loved.*

You start to feel your neck tickling. The dragon has placed a blue crystal on your throat. The crystal is the colour of the sky and makes you feel like you want to talk and tell everyone how good it feels. The dragon tells you that this crystal helps you to always speak the truth. The dragon whispers a special message: *You are honest.* You repeat, *I am honest.*

The dragon places an indigo coloured crystal on your forehead. The crystal is a beautiful deep dark blue, just like the sky at midnight. You feel very calm and still. You can't hear anything, just the quiet in your mind. The dragon whispers a special message: *I am quiet.* You repeat, *I am quiet.*

The dragon places the last crystal on your head. It is a beautiful violet colour and you watch as the violet light from the crystal spreads all over your body. It makes you feel light, as if you are a feather floating gently in the wind. The dragon whispers a special message: *You are free.* You repeat, *I am free.*

You feel so good as you discover that the crystals have made you glow in all the seven colours of the rainbow. You feel energised and balanced and thank the dragon for helping you.

Spend as long as you like in the dragon's cave and come back and see him whenever you need to. He will always be there for you with his magic crystals...

I am
balanced

Rainbow Thoughts

- *If you are feeling out of sorts sometimes it is good to sit quietly and say some positive affirmations to help you change your focus and rebalance.*

- *Colours have a wonderful way of making us feel better.*

- *Use your intuition and see which colour you need.*
  Try to visualise it and wear it.

- *Using colour can you feel balanced and re-energised.*

Spring Clean

Imagine that your brain is just like a house. It is a special two storey house with a front door a back door. On the first level it has five big bedrooms. On the second level is a very special room. Today you are going to give your brain a spring clean.

You look down and see that in your hand you have a big duster. This is not an ordinary duster. It is a magic duster and when you wave it, anything that you wish, is cleaned away. It will clean out cobwebs, wash floors, sweep up dirt and it will even make things disappear with just one wave. Your magic duster can even fix up cracks and paint walls.

You open the front door to your brain and enter with the magic duster in your hand. You look around and can see five doors. Each door is made of a different material. You walk towards the first door. It is made out of a rainbow. You notice that it is quite dull and dusty. You open the door and walk in. It is the room of vision. This is the room that helps you to see clearly. You look all around you and see that it is full of mess and much cluttered. What else can you see? You take your magic duster and clean out the room. You dust off the cobwebs and get rid of any junk that is lying around. Check the walls of your room and see if there are any cracks that need repairing or walls that need painting. You make the room neat and tidy. When you have finished, open the window to your room of vision and let it fill with fresh air and warm sunlight. How do you feel? What can you see? Can you see more clearly? You look at the rainbow door and see that it is shining very brightly and the handle is now glowing.

You now move to the second door. This door is made from a soft spongy material like a tongue. It looks very unhealthy and pale. You open the door and find that you have entered the room of taste. You take out your magic duster and clean away just as you did before. You clean out old food scraps and use your magic duster to brush and wash down all the walls until they are clean and sparkling. When you are finished you open the window and let the room fill will cool fresh air. Your tongue starts to tingle and you notice that the door knob is glowing and that the spongy door looks healthy again.

You move to the third door. This door is made from dusty strings. You open the door and realise that you have entered the room of sound. You take out your magic duster and clean away. You check the walls for cracks and holes and patch them up. You wash and clean and take away any clutter so that the room is completely empty and that it is easy for sound to enter and leave. When you have finished, open the window and fill the room with fresh clean air. You hear the most beautiful sound like a harp is playing. The breeze has made the strings on the door play and you notice the door knob glowing. Your job here is done.

The fourth door is next and you notice that it is made from smelly, runny, gooey sludge. You are very careful not to touch it as you enter. You have entered the room of smell.

You take out your magic duster and begin to work on this room. You clean and tidy and get rid of any dust and grime. You wave your duster in the air and all the awful smells disappear. When you are finished you open the window and let the fresh air in. The runny, gooey sludge is gone and the door is now covered in flowers. The beautiful smell wafts through the room. You take a deep breath in. It feels wonderful to be able to smell such wonderful smells. You close the door and notice that the door knob is now glowing. Another room is finished.

You move to the last door on this floor and notice that there is nothing there, just an empty frame. Your hand goes straight through it as if there is nothing there. You enter the room and start to clean it with your duster. As you clean away you notice that the door is beginning to appear inside the frame. It is covered with so many wonderful things for you to touch, you realise this is the room of touch. There are rough things, smooth things, spiky things, soft things. What else can you feel? Your fingers start to tingle and the more you clean the more they tingle. You open the window and let the breeze in, the door knob glows and you know it is time to move onto the final room.

You walk upstairs to the last room. The door is open and you walk in. It looks very dusty and smells very musty and old. There seems to be a lot of cobwebs in this room. As you clean you realise that the roof of this room has a huge glass dome set in it. This is the room of your inner vision. This is room you use to see with when your eyes are closed. You set your duster to work and soon the room is clean and sparkling and the dome is completely clear. You look up into the dome. What can you see? This dome is the window to your imagination.

Now that all the rooms of your senses are clean you can imagine anything you wish too. Think of something wonderful and see it created in your dome. Now see what else you can think of? Watch as the dome comes alive with all the different sights, sounds, smells, textures and tastes that your imagination has to offer.

Spend as long as you like looking through your dome. Remember that you can come back and clean these rooms any time you need to...

I have a great imagination

Rainbow Thoughts

- *Our imagination is not just visual; we use sounds, smells, feelings, texture and touch to help create images.*

- *Sometimes we need to clear our mind of the jumble so that we can take in new information or access information that we already know but just can't seem to remember.*

- *Our imagination can help us to solve problems by helping us think through different situations and their outcomes. It also helps us to think creatively.*

- *De-cluttering and clearing your bedroom also helps to clear your mind - Give it a go!*

The Rainbow Fairies

Imagine that you are out walking in the woods enjoying the fresh clean air when you come to a clearing and find a sparkling pool of water. You walk down to the water's edge and have a drink of the cool and refreshing water. You notice all the beautiful soft green grass and flowers surrounding the pool. The flowers are all the colours of the rainbow, Red, Orange, Yellow, Blue, Green, Indigo and Violet. What else can you see?

You see something move out of the corner of your eye. You look carefully at the flowers and see that sitting in the centre of each one is a tiny little fairy. These are rainbow fairies.

The fairies tell you not to be afraid and ask you to sit comfortably in the soft green grass and relax. They are going to teach you something special. They are going to teach you rainbow breathing.

A little red fairy flies over your head and sprinkles magic red fairy dust on you. You take a big breath in and breathe in the red fairy dust. You can feel the colour red spread throughout your body. You take a few more deep breaths. The fairy tells you that the colour red is energising and makes you feel fit and strong.

Next the orange fairy flies over your head and sprinkles magic orange fairy dust on you. You take a big breath in and breathe in the orange fairy dust. You can feel the colour orange spread throughout your body. You take a few more deep breaths. The fairy tells you that the colour orange makes you feel happy.

Like a small ray of sunshine the little yellow fairy comes towards you. She sprinkles yellow dust all over you. You take a big breath in and breathe in the yellow fairy dust. You can feel the colour yellow spreading throughout your body. You take a few more deep breaths. The fairy tells you that the colour yellow helps you to feel confident.

Next the tiny green fairy hovers over your head. She has glittering wings and spreads a trail of green fairy dust over you. You take a big breath in and breathe in the green fairy dust. You can feel the colour green spread throughout your body. You take a few more deep breaths. The fairy tells you that the colour green helps you to feel good about yourself.

The blue fairy flies in and sprinkles her blue dust. The dust is the colour of the sky on a bright sunny day. You take a big breath in and breathe in the blue fairy dust. You can feel the colour blue spread throughout your body. You take a few more deep breaths. The fairy tells you that the colour blue helps you to always speak the truth.

You watch as the indigo fairy comes forward. She is a beautiful dark blue and looks like the sky at midnight. She sprinkles you with her indigo dust. You take a big breath in and breathe in the indigo fairy dust. You can feel the colour indigo spread throughout your body. You take a few more deep breaths. The fairy tells you that the colour indigo helps with your imagination.

The last fairy to visit you is the violet fairy. She has beautiful violet wings speckled with white and gold. She seems to shine very brightly as she sprinkles you with violet fairy dust. You take a big breath in and breathe in the violet fairy dust. You can feel the colour violet spread throughout your body. You take a few more deep breaths. The fairy tells you that violet helps you to feel very peaceful and quiet.

You feel very balanced and calm. The fairies tell you to practice rainbow breathing whenever you need to, and you can choose one colour or all the colours of the rainbow. They tell you that you can visit any time you wish. You thank the fairies for teaching you rainbow breathing.

Spend as long as you like practising your rainbow breathing and enjoying the magic of colour...

I am peaceful and calm

Rainbow Thoughts

- *Colours are thought to have different effects on the body including healing and balancing.*
- *Breathing exercises can help to calm the body and mind quickly and easily.*
- *You can focus on just one colour when you need it for a specific purpose from the seven in the visualisation.*
- *Colours that we like and wear can tell us a lot about our personalities. List down the colours you wear a lot and research what they mean. See if this is true of your personality.*

The Rainbow Tree

Imagine that you are standing at the edge of a meadow. The meadow is high up on a mountain surrounded by beautiful, big, tall fir trees. It is a sunny morning and there are a few white clouds drifting across the sky. The sunlight gently warms your skin and you close your eyes for a few seconds and feel it dance across your face. You take a big breath in and feel the cool mountain air fill your lungs. It is so refreshing. If you look carefully you can see the top of the mountain from the meadow. Its peak seems to disappear into the clouds. What else can you see? You look around the meadow and notice that the meadow is covered with soft green grass. It looks like shaggy green carpet. You run your hands through it. How does it feel? Can you still feel the morning dew?

There are tiny white and yellow flowers scattered through out the meadow. You can also see some pink and blue ones. What else do you see in the field?

Something across the meadow catches your eye. Growing in the centre of the meadow is a magnificent tree. It is unlike anything you have ever seen before. It must have been here for hundreds of years. It has a large wooden trunk that twists and turns and it has beautiful big leaves but these leaves are not just green, -there are red leaves, blue leaves, yellow leaves and orange ones. There are also leaves in all different shades of purple. It is an amazing sight. You run towards the tree to take a better look. As you get closer to the tree you notice that where the sunlight shines upon the leaves, they appear to sparkle like tiny diamonds. It looks like hundreds of miniature rainbows.

As you get to the base of the tree you see a sign. It says,

The Rainbow Tree
You are welcome to rest beneath my leaves.
If anything is troubling you, I will set it free.
What colour do you need today?

You sit underneath the Rainbow Tree resting your back along its sturdy trunk. You instantly feel relaxed and calm. It is so cool under the leaves. You close your eyes and listen carefully. Can you hear the sound of the wind rustling the leaves? What else can you hear? You feel yourself relaxing further into the tree. The tree feels soft and welcoming, you almost feel like you are sinking into the trunk. You feel very peaceful sitting under the rainbow tree. Anything that is troubling you seems to disappear and you feel very clear and free. Any aches or pains that you have seem to vanish. You feel very happy and content.

You hear the leaves above you rustle and look up to see that the rainbow tree has changed colour. All the leaves have turned to the colour that you need for today, just as it was written on the sign. What colour do you see today? Maybe there is more than one colour?

The Rainbow Tree senses the colour that you need to feel calm and balanced. You watch as all the leaves on the rainbow tree turn to your special colour. You take some deep breaths in and think about how the colours make you feel. Listen very carefully.

What message does the rainbow tree have for you today?

Spend as long as you like walking in the meadow and relaxing under the rainbow tree. You can come back anytime you need to feel clear and balanced...

I am clear and balanced

Rainbow Thoughts

- *Sometimes if you are not feeling well or are feeling "out of sorts" just sitting quietly can help you to work out why.*
- *Red can help you feel strong, safe and secure.*
- *Orange helps you to feel happy and creative.*
- *Yellow helps you feel confident and is good for studying.*
- *Green helps you feel loved and to forgive.*
- *Blue is a peaceful colour that helps you to speak up.*
- *Indigo is great for your imagination.*
- *Violet helps you feel connected to everyone and everything and is a very relaxing colour.*
- *All together the colours of the rainbow help you to feel balanced.*

Four Seasons

Imagine that you are standing in a big white room. The room is square in shape and has no windows, just four big doors, one on each side of the room. Each door is a different colour and has a big picture painted on it. You walk forward towards the first door. This door is bright yellow and has a big sun painted on it. You open the door slowly and step through. You immediately feel how warm it is. The sun is bright and there is very little wind. You can see lots of beach sand and the glistening water of the ocean. You have entered into the season of summer.

You take a good look around you; the sky is blue and clear. What else can you see? Take a deep breath in. What does summer smell like? You walk towards the ocean. You can hear seagulls squawking and the sound of the waves as they lap against the shore. What else do you hear?

You close the door and return to the white room. This time you open the second door. This door is bright orange and has a picture of a giant leaf on the door. You open the door and step through. Your feet crunch as you walk and you see that the ground is covered in brown leaves; you realise you have stepped into autumn. Take a look around, what do you see? Can you see all the orange, yellow and brown leaves on the trees? Can you see the trees that have already lost all their leaves? You take a deep breath in. What does autumn smell like? You pick up some of the leaves with your hands and throw them into the light autumn breeze and watch them twirl and fall. You walk around for a little longer enjoying autumn and then return to the orange door. You close the door and are back in the white room.

You head towards the third door. This door is quite hard to find because it is the same colour as the room, all white. It has a picture of a snowflake on the door. This must be the door to winter. You open it and step through. You immediately feel the chilly air on your face and your nose and ears start to turn cold. You take a deep breath in. What does winter smell like? This must be a really cold winter. The ground is covered in snow, you pick some up and taste it. What does it feel like? What does it taste like?

You notice that the trees have white tips and that the top of the branches are covered in snow. What else can you see? Can you see the footprints in the snow? What animals do you think have walked through here? You feel it start to rain and decide it is time to return to the white room, splashing in the rain puddles as you go.

Once you are back in the white room, you open the last door. This door is green and has a picture of a flower painted on it. You open the door and step into spring. It is warm and the sun is shining. There are a few clouds drifting in the sky and you can see the fresh green grass and smell the beautiful perfume of flowers in the air. What else can you smell? What does spring smell like?

All the flowers are in bud and there are butterflies and bees busy at work. Can you see the birds flying from tree to tree? Look carefully into the shrubs, you may see some baby animals or birds. You run your hands through the soft green grass and walk from flower to flower smelling their scent. What else can you see on this glorious spring day?

You return to the white room and think about all the wonderful colours and changes that occur with each season and how lucky you are to be able to enjoy them.

Spend time in your favourite season, appreciating all the wonderful things that Mother Nature has to offer and come back and visit any time you wish...

I enjoy the beauty of nature

Rainbow Thoughts

- *Take time to appreciate nature and what each season brings with it.*

- *Spending time in nature is good for you both mentally and physically.*

- *Being out in nature is a great way to relieve stress and tension.*

- *Even thinking about nature and visualising being in nature can help you to relax.*

Holiday House

Imagine that are standing in a beautiful two story, wooden house. The wooden house is built on big stilts at the top of a mountain surrounded by thick forest. The house has huge glass windows and doors and has a beautiful wooden veranda the whole way around. You walk towards the big window in front of you and take a look out? What do you see? Can you see all the tree tops? It feels like you are part of the forest canopy. If you look carefully you can see down the mountain side to where the forest meets the sea. You can see the sandy white beaches and the blue water below.

You decide to go and investigate the tracks around the house that take you through the forest. Some of the tracks lead you down to the beach and some go in other directions. You pick a path and start walking. It gently winds down the mountain. You stay on the paths so you don't damage any of the plants and animals in the area. Where does the path lead you? What do you see on the way? Do you see any animals or insects? Have a look at the different varieties of plants and trees growing as you wind your way through the vegetation.

You keep walking down the path and come to a clearing. It is a wonderful lookout area with a big wooden seat. You can see the ocean and beaches for miles as well as the trees and bushland. You rest for a couple of minutes, sitting very quietly and still taking in the beautiful scene. What can you see around you? Take some deep breaths and smell the fresh clean air. Listen very carefully. What sounds can you hear? Can you hear the birds as they weave through the trees? Can you hear the wind as it gently rustles the leaves of the trees?

After a few minutes taking in the scenery, you continue down the path until you reach white sand. You have arrived at the beach. The sand is so soft and white. You take off your shoes and wriggle your toes in it. You walk down to the ocean's edge and let the cool water lap at your ankles. Do you hear the seagulls over head? Or perhaps you see a dolphin frolicking in the waves. You look back up at the house in the trees and think how lucky you are to be in this beautiful location. You continue walking along the beach and exploring the paths.

As the sun starts to set, you find your way back to the clearing and watch as the beautiful colours of the sunset fill the sky. The beautiful colours make you feel very relaxed and peaceful. You think how lucky you are to be able to enjoy this beautiful holiday house and its wonderful surrounds.

Spend as long as you like in the holiday house, enjoying the fresh forest air, the warm ocean water, the beautiful sunsets and exploring the forest paths. You can come back and visit any time you wish...

I enjoy
spending time outdoors

Rainbow Thoughts

- *We need to take notice of all the nature that is around us and learn about it so that we can fully appreciate what we have.*

- *Learn the name of five plants and five birds that are native to the area where you live. See what information you can find out about them.*

- *We can all make a difference to our environment. Think of ways you can help the environment where you live and how you are going to do it.*

- *Unless we take care of our environment it won't be around for us or future generations to enjoy.*

Green Planet

Imagine that you a sitting in a bright red rocket. You are strapped in and ready to go on a great adventure. You have been chosen to go on a mission to visit a newly discovered planet. Your rocket is on the launch pad and you can see people waving goodbye to you from below. You wave back to them.

You look around and see all the amazing controls in the rocket. There are colourful switches and dials. The captain of the rocket flicks a special red switch. You hear the countdown sequence begin: Ten, nine, eight, seven, six, five, four, three, two, one, *BLAST OFF!*

You hear the loud sound of the jets firing and you feel your rocket propelled into the air. What does it feel like? You are going very fast but you feel safe and very excited. Once you have cleared the earth's atmosphere you look out of the window. You can see the earth below you. It is an amazing sight. Can you see the oceans? What continents can you see? You see stars twinkling in the deep blue sky. You see what looks like pockets of dense white mist.

After a short time you feel your rocket start to slow down and change direction. It is heading for a landing on a new planet. You look out the window and see that it looks much like our planet does. There are rivers and lakes and you can see mountains and hills and lots of greenery. There is so much greenery that is looks like the whole planet is green. Perhaps this is how it got the name *Green Planet.*

Your rocket ship lands with a slight bump. You hear the engines power down and wait as the door opens. You walk outside the door and see a big sign saying *Welcome to Green Planet.* Waiting to greet you are the inhabitants of Green Planet, the Nature Sprites. You have trouble seeing them at first because they are so small. The Nature Sprites are tiny little people. They are only as big as your hand. They are all dressed in flowing robes of green and brown. They have beautiful glittery gold and silver wings. They are very gentle and loving and you feel very safe with them.

They invite you to come and visit their planet. You look around and see that it looks much like planet earth would have looked a long time ago. There are no buildings or roads and there are no houses. The whole planet is in its natural state. The Nature Sprites live in little homes made of sticks that hang high in the trees. They almost look like little bird houses. Can you see them?

The Nature Sprites tell you that everything on their planet comes from the planet and is reusable. There is no rubbish on the green planet. They recycle everything and only use solar power. They tell you that they grow their own food and grains, there is no packaging and definitely nothing made of plastic on their planet. They collect rainwater for their baths and showers. They only have short showers and even collect their washing and shower water to use on their gardens.

You follow your new friends a little further. They show you their fields full of native flowers. They show you their orchards and their vegetable gardens. What can you see growing in the fields? What can you see growing in the orchards and gardens? What colours are they? You can pick a piece of fruit if you like. What does it taste like? Take a sniff of the clean fresh air and see what smells you can identify. Now the Nature Sprites take you to visit their worm farms. How many worms can you count? The Nature Sprites tell you that the worms help to break down food scraps and to make fertiliser for the vegetable garden. The Nature Sprites ask you to think about some things you can do to help make planet earth greener. You think about the changes you will make when you return to earth.

Spend as long as you like visiting the Green planet, when you are ready the Nature Sprites will take you back to your rocket for your journey home...

I think of ways I can **help** our planet

Rainbow Thoughts

- *Everything we do has an impact on the planet.*
- *Even the smallest things we do to help can make a big difference, such as picking up rubbish.*
- *We can help change the future, spend some time researching ways to help save our planet and make it greener.*
- *Find five things you can do in your home or school to make a difference.*

World of Colour

Imagine that you are sitting outside in a park. It is a beautiful day and the sky is blue. You notice a few white fluffy clouds drifting by. You can feel the sun gently tickling your face. There is a gentle breeze blowing and you can feel the soft cool grass beneath your feet.

You listen carefully. You can hear birds nearby in the trees and some off in the distance. What else can you hear?

You take a deep breath in. What can you smell? Perhaps you can smell flowers in a nearby garden bed? As you are sitting and enjoying the park you feel a light sprinkle of rain start to land on you. You realise it is a sun shower. You close your eyes and let the rain land on your face and body. It feels warm and is very relaxing. As the rain gradually stops, you open your eyes and see a giant rainbow. The rainbow seems to start at your feet.

You touch the rainbow and notice that stairs appear inside it which lead up to a door. You decide to investigate. You walk up the stairs and open the door. You see a sign saying *Welcome to the World of Colour*. You open the door and step in. As you look around you realise you have stepped on to some form of escalator and it is going to take you through the rainbow.

First you pass through the colour red. It feels warm and you feel very safe. You watch as the red light bathes you. Next you pass through orange. This colour makes you laugh and feel happy. Lots of good ideas come to you when you are in the orange light. Now you come to yellow. The yellow makes you feel confident and quite powerful. Now you pass through the soft green light. The green light makes you feel very balanced and filled with lots of love and hope. It is very calming in the green light. Now you pass through blue. The blue light makes your throat tickle and you feel like you have lots of good things to talk about. Next you pass through the dark blue light of Indigo. The indigo light sparks your imagination, and you seem to know the answers to questions when you are in the Indigo Light. Finally you reach the violet light. The violet light makes you feel very calm and very, very peaceful. You feel very clear in violet light.

Now your escalator will take you back through the colours to the start. Think about whether you need to stop at any particular colour or colours? If you want to stop just say the word *stop* and the escalator will let you relax in that colour for a few minutes.

When you are ready to leave, go back to the door, walk down the stairs and you will find yourself back in the park feeling very balanced and calm.

Spend as long as you like enjoying the world of colour. You may come back and visit any time you wish...

I enjoy the
healing power of colour

Rainbow Thoughts

- *Rainbows are one of nature's most beautiful effects.*

- *Rainbows are often used as a symbol of inner peace and harmony throughout the world.*

- *Think about what your favourite colours are and how they make you feel.*

- *Think about which colour you may need.*

Rainbow Pool

Imagine that you are standing in a beautiful rainforest. You look around and see giant green trees with wet shiny leaves. There are lush ferns and vines that wrap gently around them. What else can you see? Can you see the beautiful flowers in bright oranges, reds and yellows? Perhaps you can see the white blossoms scattered across the rainforest floor. There are butterflies and birds. Can you see the brightly coloured beetles? The rainforest is full of life today. What noises can you hear in the rainforest? You take a deep breath in and let your lungs fill with this clean, fresh air. The air is warm and moist. There is a beautiful scent in the air? See if you can identify it.

Ahead, in the distance, you can see something sparkling. You walk towards it and as you get closer you see the sparkles are sunlight dancing on a beautiful pool of water. The water is so still and clear that is looks like a mirror. You sit beside the pool of water and stare into your reflection. As you stare you notice that the water is changing colours. First it changes to red, then orange, yellow and green. It changes to blue, then deep purple and a soft violet. You have found a magical rainbow pool.

You sit watching the colours as they continue to change through all the colours of the rainbow. It is so beautiful to watch and has a very calming effect. You put your finger in the pool and something amazing happens. The colour spreads from the pool, up you finger and over your whole body until you are completely covered in the colour. You look down at yourself and every single part of you is that colour. The rainbow pools seem to know what colour you need today. Look carefully. What colour is it telling you that you need? It may be several colours. You keep taking deep breaths and relaxing by the rainbow pool enjoying being your colour. You will know you are finished once the rainbow pool returns to looking like a mirror.

You thank the rainbow pool for helping you .You feel very balanced and refreshed. All your aches and pains have disappeared and it feels like anything that was worrying or upsetting you has gone. You feel re energised, healthy and full of positive energy. It is a wonderful feeling.

Spend as long as you like enjoying the rainforest and the healing powers of the rainbow pool. You can return whenever you wish...

Amazing things
happen to me
every day

Rainbow Thoughts

- *Draw daily inspiration from nature and life.*
  There is nothing more inspiring than a rainbow in the sky.

- *There is magic all around us.*
  We just need to open our eyes and take notice.

- *Listen carefully when you are outside and count how many sounds you can hear.*

- *Sit and observe when you are outside and count how many different forms of life there are.*

- *If you think amazing things will happen every day, then you are sure to attract them.*

- *The most amazing thing can be as simple as seeing a flower open that was just a little bud the day before.*

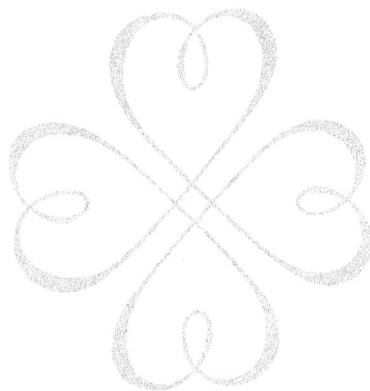

MEDITATION AND RELAXATION
FOLLOW-UP ACTIVITIES

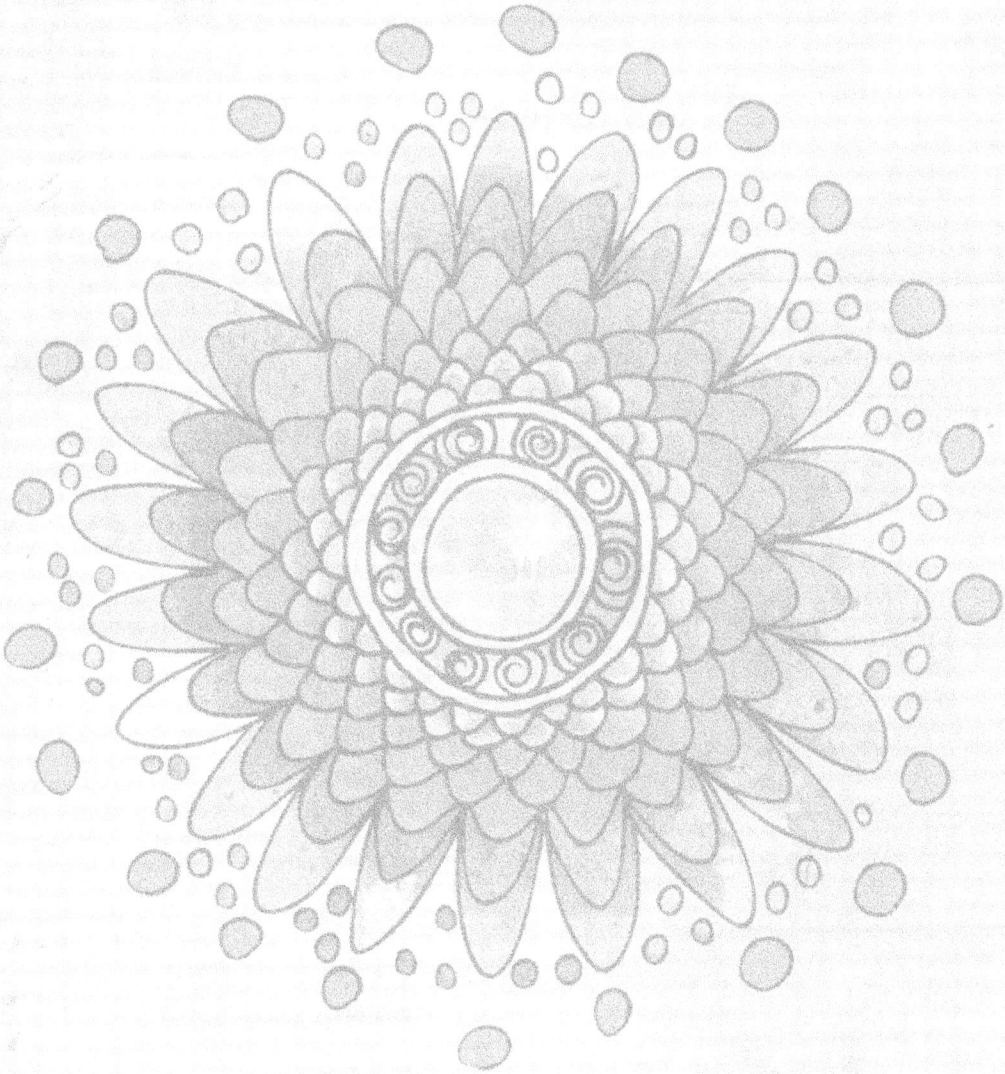

Poems

Drama

Collage

Sharing

Writing

Journal

Painting

Drawing

Sculpture

Follow-up
Activities

Make Music

Arts & Crafts

Clay Modelling

Creative Dance

Meditation and Relaxation Follow-up Activities

I am continually in awe of young children and how quickly they slip into a relaxed state and the amazing discussions that come after meditation or relaxation sessions. Some of the artwork and journal entries that I have seen produced from their journeys are incredible and inspirational. Children tend to be very creative and expressive following a meditation or relaxation session. Creative activities help to balance and ground a child. They also help to express and reinforce the inner journey to the outer journey.

Here are a few activities that can be done at home or in a class situation to follow up after a meditation session or they can be done on their own as another avenue to foster self-confidence, awareness and gratitude. A large proportion of the activities are centred on colour which can be a very good tool for children to use as part of relaxation and meditation. I have mostly written the activities as if in a classroom setting but the activities can easily be adjusted for home. Some of the activities in this section are repeated from *Indigo Dreaming- Meditations for Children* as a reminder and to reinforce their use following a meditation or relaxation session.

The activities have been broken up into:

- General Activities
- Colour Activities
- Rainbow Activities

> **Your imagination is your preview of life's coming attractions.**
> *Albert Einstein*

General Activities

Questions

Once your meditation session is over one of the best things you can do is give children time to reflect and then prompt them with some questions. I find that having a big piece of paper ready for children to write or draw on helps. As children get older they often self reflect without any prompting. Give them a few minutes to draw or write. Then prompt with questions such as; how did you feel? What did you see? What did you smell? What sounds did you hear? They can then share as below.

Discussion/Sharing Circle

As above, ask the child to reflect on what they experienced. They can then share their experiences with each other. You can do a discussion and sharing following the meditation, in pairs or small groups or have a sharing circle. Reinforce that there are no interruptions or judgements when someone is sharing. It is important to understand that everyone's experiences will be different and that they are all equally important and valid. You may need to prompt them to begin with i.e. Did they see, hear or feel anything? What ideas came to them? Do they feel refreshed? What colours did they see?

The meditation may have been chosen as part of a topic, issue or theme. This will provide a starting discussion point and allow children to share their feelings. Also keep in mind that some children may not wish to discuss their meditation and let them know that this is okay.

Creative Writing

After doing a meditation or relaxation exercise, get children to write down what they experienced or any ideas that came to them. They can do it in a journal or on paper.

Using visualisation before writing a story or poem can help a child open the door to their imagination. For example, if you are writing a poem or story about the beach, you can ask the children to close their eyes and take a few deep breaths. Then ask them to imagine they are at the beach, ask them what it smells like, what it feels like, what they can see and what they can hear. Give them a minute or so to visualise before they open their eyes. They can them begin their exercise. Wonderful stories and wordplay will emerge as the child has had a chance to experience what they are about to write. Rather than being a distant scene, they have actually participated in the scene, and experienced it.

Artwork

Following a meditation, children can draw, paint or make a collage based on what they experienced and visualised. Children can make sculptures out of clay or paper mache. I often hear children say that their great ideas just came to them when they were relaxed. Meditation and Relaxation can lead into many different types of art activities. This will provide a colourful and very positive classroom or bedroom.

Meditation Scrapbook or Journal

Children can make their own meditation scrapbook or journal. After each meditation or relaxation session, ask your child to draw what they saw and write down any words, thoughts or ideas that came to them. They can draw pictures, cut and paste pictures, write affirmations and generally express their thoughts and feelings. It is interesting to see how the child develops as they participate in more visualisation and relaxing activities and they are a great insight into their thoughts and feelings. Older children may like to write their own visualisations. Parents or teachers may need to help. You can start it with *Imagine....* These can then be tried at home or in class.

Children can also add any favourite quotes, sayings, affirmations, inspiring stories, relaxing scenes or pictures they resonate with. I have had children stick gum leaves, dried flowers and even beach sand sprinkled on glue into their journals and scrapbooks. Children love working with textures and smells.

Gratitude Journal

Another great use for a meditation scrapbook or journal is to have a gratitude section. After each day or for each entry, children can write 3 things for which they are grateful. It can be things like; my comfortable bed at night, my friend Lisa etc. It is a good habit for children to get into and helps with positive talk. Start it off with *Today I am grateful for...*

Worry Hat

You can make a big Magic Worry Hat out of cardboard with your child/children. This can be put in their bedroom or in the classroom. The child can write down anything that is worrying them and pin it to the Magic Worry Hat. This can then be discussed or a meditation chosen to help with the issue. The Worry Hat can also be used as mini-meditation in its own right. Children can visualise the hat, then visualise putting it on and then imagine that all their worries are drifting up from their head into the hat and that they now feel clear and calm. This is a good activity to do to start the day or when a child is feeling anxious or confused. Remind the child that they can use their Magic Worry Hat at any time. (Note: This can also be done as a Worry Tree).

Magic Shield

Children can make their Magic Shield from the *Peaceful Warrior* visualisation. They can be given an array of different materials to create it. These look fantastic displayed in the classroom or bedroom.

I am Collage

You will need magazines, glue, scissors and cardboard for this activity. Each child will need a big piece of paper or cardboard with **I AM** written at the top in big bold letters. They can then scour the magazines and cut out words that fit with I am, such as; *happy, amazing, friendly, talented*, and paste them on the page until it is full. This makes a great poster for display in class or in a child's bedroom to reinforce positive qualities and remind them that they are special.

Gratitude Jar

This is a great visual activity. Each child will need a jar or you can make a huge jar for the class. You will need something small that you can place in the jar and count with such as pebbles, nuts, counters, beads, marbles, glass beads, feathers, buttons or you can cut out pieces of cardboard and write on them. Everyday you must think of something you are grateful for and place a pebble, nut etc into the jar to represent it. If you use cardboard you can actually write on it what you are grateful for. Continue this everyday until the jar is full. Then discuss how many things there are to be grateful for and that sometimes we forget this. It is a great way for children to get into the habit of expressing gratitude everyday.

This activity can also be done as an Affirmation Jar. You can help your child with an affirmation that is relevant at the time. Each day say the affirmation i.e. *I am strong and healthy*, and place a marble or another object in the jar. Once the jar is full go on to your new affirmation. They say it takes a minimum of 21 days to change behaviour and to make it automatic in the conscious mind, so this is a great way to keep count and to get those positive thoughts and expectations flowing.

Making a Mantra

This activity can be done as a class or on an individual basis. Think of a goal or area that you would like to improve on or have a more positive outlook about. Work on a positive statement, sentence or affirmation that becomes your mantra, for example *I am strong and powerful, I practice acts of kindness every day, I will do more to care for the environment, I can do it, I will try all new things that come my way with a good attitude*. Write your mantra down and then decorate it. For a class you can make a massive banner and hang it or a large wall poster. For home you can make a poster or banner that hangs across the window. Try and repeat it at least 5 times a day, especially first thing in the morning.

Relaxation Box

This is a similar concept to the affirmation box. It can also be done as a board or poster if that resonates better with you or your child. Find a box and decorate it with relaxing pictures such as beach scenes. You can also add relaxing affirmations and words to it. Inside the box you can place all the tools you need to relax. Some of the things you can add include:

- Pictures or scenes that you can look at that feel relaxing, cut them out of magazines and place them on cardboard.
- Any objects you use for relaxation i.e. stress ball, tennis ball for massaging your feet, eye pillow, sea shell, essential oil.
- Any inspiring messages, quotes, affirmations or words. Write them out and place them in the box.

Now when you need to do some relaxation you have your box ready. Look through your box and begin to relax!

What Makes Me Grow?

I love doing this activity with children. It has been adapted from a school health education activity and is a lot of fun for adults and children to do. Normally when you buy a packet of seeds or a plant they come with information or a label saying how to take care of them and the instructions for use. Example "plant 10cm apart, likes part sun, fertilise regularly" and so on. The idea for this activity is to get everyone to make their own seed packet.

You will need a piece of cardboard to make a giant seed packet or plant label. Fold the cardboard in half and glue or staple up the sides and the bottom, leave the top open. Children can then decorate the front with their name and picture. On the back they can list all the instructions to help them to grow as a person i.e. "How to make (child's name) grow". Ask them to think of things they need to make them feel happy, safe, loved and relaxed. For example: needs lots of hugs, likes watching sunsets, loves the colour blue, needs to spend quiet time reading each day, doesn't like loud noise...

In addition to this, if you leave the top of the packet open i.e. not glued or stapled they can be filled with *seeds*. These seeds can be pieces of paper or cardboard with affirmations, goals or dreams written on them. In a class situation you can have students make a seed with something nice written on it for someone else to place it in their packet.

These look great hanging in classroom on a string with flowers and leaves in between or you can display them on a stick in a painted pot filed with soil. Children can also cut out leaves to attach to the stick and surround the packet with a flower or vegetable cut out.

Colour Activities

Colour is everywhere around us and is a big part of everyday life. We use colour in our homes to decorate and express ourselves. Colour is in the foods we eat and the clothes we wear. Nature provides us with a brilliant array of colours in flowers, plants, animals, insects, trees, rainbows and much more.

We often use colour in our everyday speech to describe the emotions we are feeling such as; green with envy, seeing red, having a grey day, and feeling blue. Without colour our lives would very be dull and non descript. Making children aware of colour helps with different aspects of the visualisation process and helps to provide a tool for balancing their bodies.

Research on colour

Get students to do some research on colour. You can ask some of the following questions;

- What is your favourite colour?
- Which colours don't you like?
- Discuss how different colours make you feel.
- What colour is mostly in your wardrobe?
- What colours are in your home?
- What are your family members' favourite colours?
- What are primary and secondary colours?
- Which colours are warm colours?
- Which are cool colours?
- Which are neutral colours?
- How many colours are there?
- Can we see all colours?
- What colours make you feel calm?

Older students can research how colours are used in the everyday work places such as hospitals or restaurants according to their properties. For example, red is meant to stimulate the appetite and is often used in restaurants. Pale green is a calming colour that is associated with healing so it is often used in hospitals. They can research colours used in company logos and the colours used by fast food outlets. Research how we use colour in everyday speech and associations, for example, green with envy. Look at the colours that are used in traffic lights. There are many interesting projects that involve colour.

Research Colour Healing

Get students to discuss how colours are used in healing. Discuss how some people feel better wearing a certain coloured garment. Look at visualising a colour, placing coloured material over an affected body part, using colour breathing, sleeping on a pillow case of that colour etc. This is a great class activity done in groups. You can give each group a different colour of the rainbow and see what they can discover.

Colour Weeks

You can organise a colour week for your class or at home and follow the theme through all activities. For example, if it is red week you can ask the children to wear the colour red. You can read stories based on the colour red, for example, 'The Little Red Engine'. You can discuss foods of that colour and maybe try some of them. You can make collages of that colour using magazines and other items. You can then continue the discussion about which were their favourite colours and how each colour made them feel.

Creating Colours

You will need some paint in trays or on ice-cream lids and some brushes and paper. Using the three primary colours of red, blue and yellow children can experiment and mix colours to see what colours they can make. What happens when you add black and white to colours? This can lead on to a discussion of shades and tints.

Colour Wheel

The children will need to draw a circle on card or paper and cut it out. Divide the circle into 6 parts. Colour in three of the sections of circle red, yellow and blue (make sure there is a section in between each). Now colour in the secondary colours in the remaining sections. Secondary colours are the colours you make when you mix the primary colours (red and yellow have orange in between, yellow and blue have green and red and blue have purple in between). Children can then discuss the colours and you can talk about complimentary colours. The complimentary colour is the colour opposite on the wheel i.e. blue's complimentary colour is orange. You can extend this activity by doing a 12-section wheel by continuing to mix the colours above.

Crystals

Children love crystals. There are so many different crystals and gems of all different colours. Ask children to research a crystal. They can discuss where it comes from and what special properties it has. Do certain colour crystals have similar properties? For example, Rose Quartz is a pink crystal and is good to place by your bed at night to help with peaceful dreams and is a lovely crystal to give someone who is feeling sad. It is readily found throughout the world. Research the different parts of the world they come from and how rare are they? For example, Bloodstone is readily found in countries such as Australia, Brazil and China and is meant to be able to help cleanse the blood and is good for increasing creativity.

Mandalas

Children love creating and colouring Mandalas. Mandalas are a configuration of geometric figures or shapes that are said to symbolise the universe. They are seen as a symbol or unity and wholeness and involve a circle shape. Mandalas are great for concentration and focus and are very relaxing to do.

Children can create a Mandala of their own or colour in one that has been designed. There are some great Mandala's and resources on this fantastic website *www.papermandalas.com.* If children are creating their own Mandala you can discuss that they are making a special circle. They then fill them with patterns, shapes and colours. Circles can be cut out of cardboard or drawn on paper then just let the creativity flow. They will need crayons, textas or pencils. They can be simple or complex, it is totally up to the child. Older children may like to use drawing equipment to make geometric designs inside. Younger children may wish to draw things in their Mandala that make them happy. They can make a beautiful display at home or in a classroom.

Mandalas can also be used as a focus for meditation. Children can take some deep breaths then focus on the Mandala. Encourage them to let their mind relax and to focus on the image. It should not be done so that the child has to strain. They can do this for a few minutes and see how they feel afterwards.

Rainbow Activities

Rainbows are spectacular natural phenomena that occur when the sun shines onto droplets of moisture in the earth's atmosphere. The traditional rainbow is that made up of seven colours - red, orange, yellow, green, blue, indigo, and violet. Rainbows are actually made up of the whole continuum of colours from red to violet and colours beyond what the eye can see. The colours of the rainbow have a magical quality to them and rainbows seem to draw an inner response from everyone who experiences them.

Spiritually, rainbows are said to be a sign that everyone is going to be alright and that we are all blessed. The colours of the rainbow are used in many visualisations and healing practices throughout the world.

Research

Research what rainbows are and how they are made. See if you can find out what a double rainbow is?

Make a Handprint Rainbow

The handprints of children can be put together to make a beautiful rainbow to decorate the classroom wall or for home. For a class you will need to join several pieces of paper together to make a large rainbow, at home a piece of A3 size paper will work well. Draw an arc with seven sections. Prepare seven trays of paint, each a colour of the rainbow. Children can place their hands in a tray of paint then place them in the corresponding arc until it is covered with handprints. Repeat this for each colour until finished. This makes a great class decoration or can be done at home using a smaller sheet of paper and one finger instead of the whole hand.

Make a Paper Collage Rainbow

Draw a rainbow shape on some white paper. Children can then trace it or draw one of their own. Remind the children to draw seven arcs like a rainbow. Children can then use pieces of coloured tissue paper, sequins, buttons, feathers or any other craft material and glue them in corresponding seven arcs to create all the colours of the rainbow. Children can make their own pot of gold at the end of the rainbow or write a special rainbow wish.

Make Rainbow Flags

Cut out some small flags and make each one a different colour of the rainbow. You can make them out of cardboard or material. On each coloured flag ask the children to write a value, empowering word or positive quality that they admire i.e. joy, kindness, love, peace, sharing or calm. You can research colours and some of their associated qualities such as orange for creativity or blue for harmony. They can decorate them with borders, pictures, or icons and make them stand out using glitter or other textures. You can then join the flags on a length of string or ribbon and hang them in bedrooms or classrooms. They make a beautiful display and reinforce positive values.

Rainbow Mobiles

Children can use paint, crayons, chalks or any other drawing medium to make paper rainbows and decorate them. String them together with paper clouds or cotton wool to make a beautiful display. You can hang them on wire hangers and make a magical mobile.

Fruit Loops Rainbow

Use Fruit Loops cereal and glue to make a rainbow on a piece of paper. This is a great tactile exercise and looks fantastic. Draw the rainbow and then fill in the colours by sticking the fruit loops of the same colour together to makes the colours of the rainbow.

Rainbow Necklaces

Use coloured macaroni or beads to make a necklace or bracelet with all the colours of the rainbow. Coloured macaroni or beads can also be used to decorate pictures or paintings of rainbows.

Blow Bubbles

Blow bubbles in the sunlight and look for the rainbows to appear on them.

Making your own Rainbows

You can use glass prisms or crystals and hold them into the light and make rainbows on the wall. Children love doing this activity.

Another great activity that requires a little bit of set-up but is lots of fun is making a rainbow in a dish. You will need milk, dish detergent (make sure it is not coloured) a flat low bowl or baking dish and red, blue and yellow food colouring. Poor a cup of milk into the bowl. At one edge of the bowl put 3-4 drops of red food colouring in. Very carefully repeat this with both other colours making sure that they are evenly spread around the bowl. Be careful not to bump or move the bowl. Now squeeze some dish detergent into the middle of the dish or bowl and see what happens. You will see that the milk and detergent do not mix and the detergent spreads over the surface of the milk picking up all the different colours making the colours of the rainbow as it goes.

> If there is light in the soul,
> There will be beauty in the person.
> If there is beauty in the person,
> There will be harmony in the house.
> If there is harmony in the house,
> There will be order in the nation.
> If there is order in the nation,
> There will be peace in the world.
>
> *Chinese Proverb*

When we are unable to find tranquility

within ourselves,

it is useless to seek it elsewhere.

Francois de La Rochefoucauld

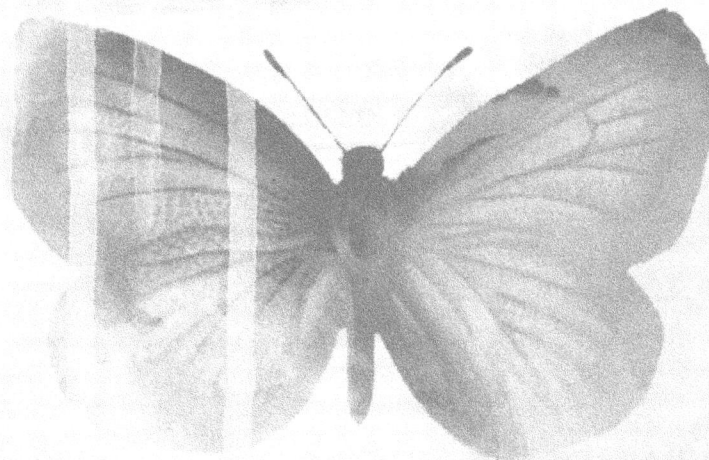

Conclusion

Serenity is inside all of us, and we just need to know how to tap into it. We can teach our children how to find this place of peace and learn to cope in our ever changing world. We can teach our children how to listen to their hearts and trust their own intuition. We can teach our children to be compassionate, loving and forgiving and to understand their emotions and feelings. We can teach them to let their imaginations run free and to explore their creativity. We can help them to have experiences and enjoy pastimes that are not always part of the electronic world. Let's help our children to create a simple life where they understand that possessions don't make you happy.

By learning to calm themselves children will be able to learn more effectively and to be more resilient. Our children can grow to be happy, calm and confident, totally aware of the environment in which they live and how to take care of it.

Add to this a healthy diet, exercise and a good dose of outdoor and imaginative play and we are giving our children the best chance to cope with this rapid social change and the increasing pressures placed upon them.

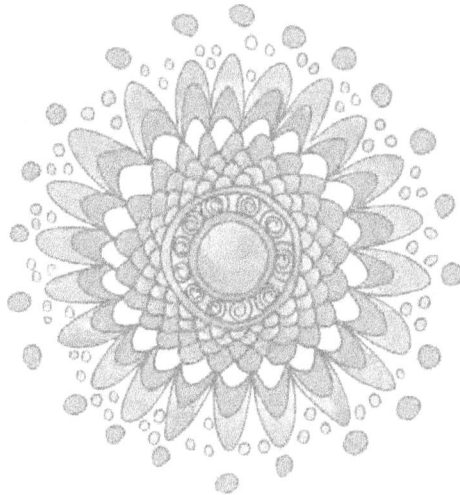

INDEX OF VISUALISATIONS AND ACTIVITIES

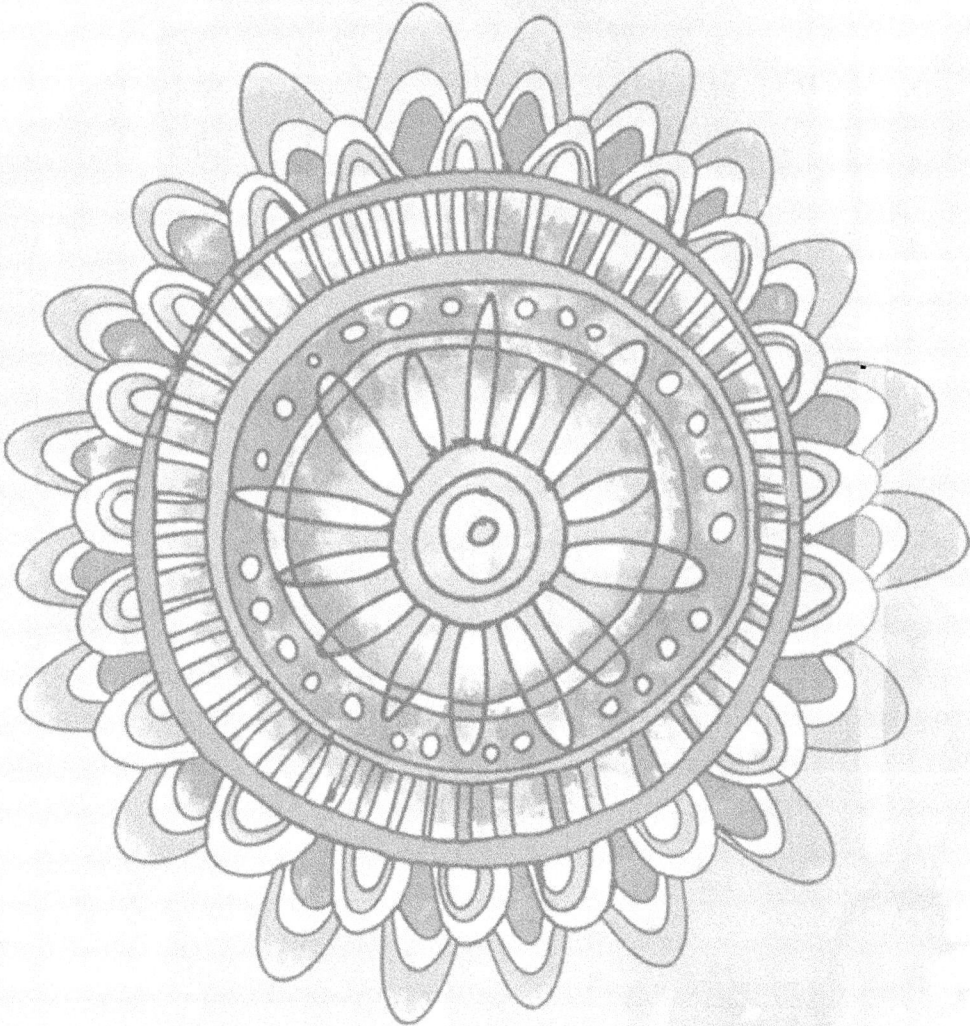

Quick Find Index of Visualisations

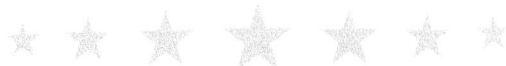

★ ★ ★ ★ ★ ★ ★

Quick Find Index of Visualisations by Value/Issue

RESOURCES

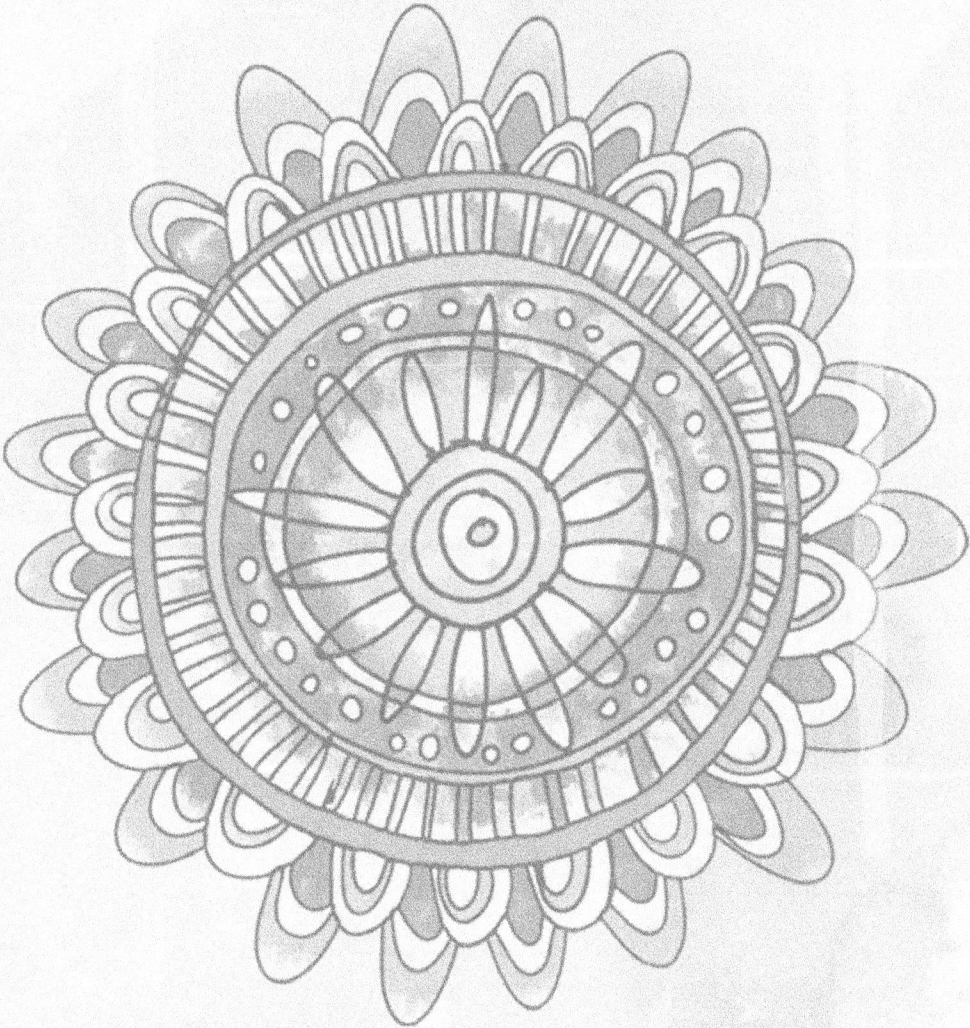

Resources

Here are some of my favourite resources. I have also listed some references for adults who wish to read more about Meditation and Visualisation.

Children Meditation and Visualisation

Moonbeam	Maureen Garth
Earthlight	Maureen Garth
Starbright	Maureen Garth
Small Souls	Roxanne Paynter
Sensational Meditation for Children	Sarah Wood Vallely
Teaching Meditation to Children	David Fontana and Ingrid Slack
Creative Visualization with Children	Jennifer Day
Meditation in Schools-Calmer Classrooms	Clive and Jane Erricker, Gina Levete
Spinning Inward	Maureen Murdock

Adults Meditation and Visualisation

The Quiet	Paul Wilson
More Quiet	Paul Wilson
A Piece of Quiet	Paul Wilson
Learn to Meditate	David Fontana
Creative Meditation and Visualization	David Fontana
Do You Want to Meditate?	Eric Harrison
Hurry up and Meditate	David Michie
Creative Visualization	Shakti Gawain
Creative Visualization for Beginners	Richard Webster

Yoga/Massage

Massage Stories for Children	Tricia Riordan
Fly Like a Butterfly: Yoga for Children	Shakta Kaur Khalsa
Who Am I?: Yoga for Children of all Ages	Jane Lee Wiesner

Nutrition and Food Additives

Chemical Free Kids	Dr Sarah Lantz PhD
Additive Alert	Julie Eady
The Chemical Maize	Bill Statham
Changing Habits Changing Lives	Cyndi O'Meara
Clean	Alejandro Junger, M.D .
Sweet Poison	David Gillespie

Aromatherapy and Wellbeing

Like Chocolate for Women	Kim Morrison and Fleur Welligan
About Face	Kim Morrison and Fleur Welligan
Like an Apple a Day	Kim Morrison and Fleur Welligan

Environment/Nature

Green is Good: Smart Ways to Live Well and Help the Planet	Rebecca Blackburn
True Green Kids	Kim McKay and Jenny Bonnin
Last Child in the Woods	Richard Louv

The Nature Principle	Richard Louv

Chemicals/Toxins in the Home

Healthy Home Healthy Family	Nicola Bijlsma
Chemical Free Home	Robin Stewart
Home Safe Home	Debra Lynn Dadd

Parenting

More Secrets of Happy Children	Steve Biddulph

Recycling/Simple Living/Living Sustainably

Down to Earth - A Guide to Simple Living	Rhonda Hetzel
down-to-earth.blogspot.com.au	
justlikemynanmade.bogspot.com.au	
slowlivingessentials.blogspot.com	

Minimalism Books and Blogs

The Simple Guide to a Minimalist Life	Leo Babauta
The Everyday Minimalist	www.everydayminimalist.com

Crystals

The Crystal Bible	Judy Hall

Research Papers and Articles

For a full list of research papers and articles please visit **www.indigokidz.com.au**

Other Products Available

Indigo Dreaming - A Book of Meditations for Children
Indigo Dreaming - Meditations for Children CD
Indigo Dreaming - Positive Affirmation Cards for Children
Indigo Dreaming - A Magical Bedtime Story Book for Children
The Rainbow in Me - Chakra Poster for Children
The Affirmation Garden - An Empowering Story Book for Children
The Affirmation Garden - Meditations and Affirmations for Children CD
Oofoo Learns to Relax - A Picture Book that Teaches Children Ways to Deal with Stress
Rainbow Dreaming - Power Thought Cards for Children

Visit us at **www.indigokidz.com.au**

Like us on Facebook at **https://www.facebook.com/indigokidzaus**

Follow us on Instagram @ **indigo_kidz**

www.ingramcontent.com/pod-product-compliance
Lightning Source LLC
Chambersburg PA
CBHW080248030426

42334CB00023BA/2742